Normalise feeling

'NOT OKAY'

in pregnancy

AF518093

Normalise feeling 'NOT OKAY' in pregnancy

Richa Kumari

Bigfoot Publications

Because, there's a writer in everyone.

Normalise feeling 'NOT OKAY' in pregnancy
Author : Richa Kumari

First Published by
Bigfoot06 Publications (OPC) Pvt. Ltd.
1st floor, BSR Building near Vishal Mega Mart,
Daultabad Flyover, Laxman Vihar Phase 3,
Gurugram, Haryana (122001)
Website: www.bigfootpublications.in
Email: info@bigfootpublications.in

First Edition : September, 2023
© Richa Kumari

ISBN Print Book - **978-81-19512-33-1**

All rights reserved. No part of this book may be reproduced or transmitted in any form or by any means, electronic or mechanical, including photocopying, recording, or by an information storage and retrieval system—except by a reviewer who may quote brief passages in a review to be printed in a magazine, newspaper, or on the Web—without permission in writing from the copyright owner.

Although the author and publisher have made every effort to ensure the accuracy and completeness of information contained in this book, we assume no responsibility for errors, inaccuracies, omissions, or any inconsistencies herein. Any slights on people, places, or organizations are unintentional.

Printed in India

DEDICATION

To the Unwavering Pillar of Strength,

In the tapestry of life's journey, there are certain souls who illuminate our path with unwavering light. To my dearest husband, whose unwavering support and boundless love have been the cornerstone of my journey through pregnancy and beyond.

As I penned the stories of these incredible women and their battles, triumphs, and transformative moments, I was reminded of the unspoken camaraderie that underpins every powerful journey. Your steadfast presence, endless patience, and unyielding encouragement have been my sanctuary during the most profound time of my life.

In your arms, I found solace in moments of uncertainty. Your understanding heart held space for my emotions as they ebbed and flowed with the tides of pregnancy. Your belief in me and in the strength of the stories I chose to share ignited the spark of determination within me.

Through these tales, I hope to illuminate not only the power of a woman's journey but also the resonance of a partnership that empowers and uplifts. To you, my partner in everything, my confidante, and my greatest source of strength–this book is dedicated with a heart brimming with gratitude and love.

With you by my side, every word, every page, and every story comes alive in a symphony of shared dreams and unwavering support. Here's to the journey we've walked together and the stories we continue to create–one beautiful chapter at a time.

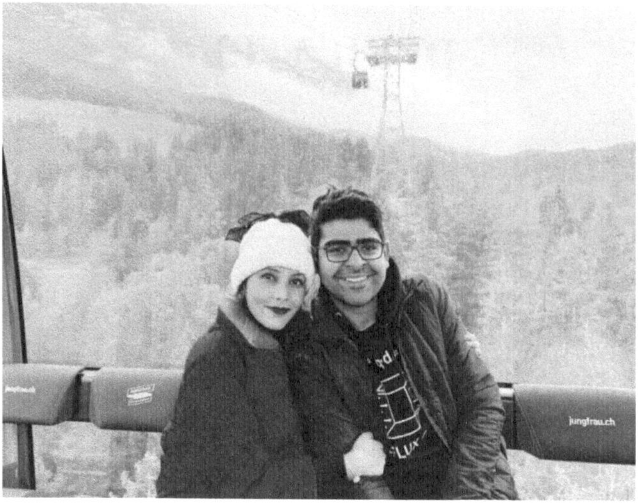

PREFACE

Within the pages of this captivating book lies the enthralling tales of nine remarkable pregnant women whose lives were forever changed by the power of support, spread across nine different chapters representing the nine months of pregnancy. As we step into the vibrant tapestry of modern society, we are beckoned not only to empower women but also to embrace the presence of empowered women as a transformative force.

In this enchanting journey, we meet Sagarika in Chapter 1, a woman determined to shatter the chains of orthodox beliefs held by her mother-in-law, all in the pursuit of savoring the full spectrum of joy that pregnancy brings. Alongside her stands Samiksha Tiwari in chapter 2, whose path is marred by the constant scrutiny of her boss, igniting a fire to rise above judgment and emerge stronger.

Then in chapter 3, Divya's heart whispers a yearning for her husband to delve into the depths of her emotions, longing for an unspoken connection that transcends words. In chapter 4, Richa's story unfurls as she strives to convey to her closest confidantes the profound metamorphosis that pregnancy truly entails—a journey of raw transformation, not just a fleeting event.

Venturing further, we meet Parvartika in chapter 5, ensnared by the enigmatic allure of social media, trapped in the whirlwind of others' lives while longing to traverse her own path. In the next chapter, Raghavi's world is cast into a web of misinterpretation, her husband misconstruing the sage advice of her doctor, leading her onto an unforeseen path.

Intrigue deepens as Alka's narrative emerges—a career-driven woman who grapples with the sacrifices of pregnancy, a tale of striking a balance amidst the storm. The subsequent pages resonate with the enigmatic tale of contrasting choices: the stories of Parineeta and Lavanya, where the veiled narratives of c-section and natural delivery cast their shadows.

But the journey doesn't end there; it delves into the uncharted territories of the postpartum realm through the eyes of Beena—a woman navigating the labyrinth of new motherhood, her aspirations and expectations intertwining with her reality.

Step into this world where the threads of these women's lives intertwine with the universal experience of pregnancy. Their stories beckon, inspire, and evoke empathy, inviting you to explore the intricate nuances of life's most awe-inspiring journey—motherhood.

At the end, it is important to prioritise the mental health over everything else. The book is going to talk about 'it is okay not being okay'.

PROLOGUE

This book has a purpose: it wants to help us openly address the challenges we face and create a world where we can have real, honest conversations. It underlines the importance of building a society where women can not only openly express their needs but also get the support they deserve.

In today's world, we often hide our true feelings to show a more positive image of our lives. This leads us to forget that we're all human, with both joys and sorrows. Unfortunately, the current trend involves posting on social media, avoiding genuine conversations, and hiding our emotions. This results in us living in a shallow and untruthful way.

This book encourages you to step out of your comfort zone and talk about practical ways to handle pregnancy. It reminds us that pregnancy is a natural process, not a sickness, but it should also not be trivialized. We need to understand the complex emotions that pregnant women may hide behind their smiles.

If you strongly hold traditional beliefs or value the authenticity that social media lacks, this book may not be the right fit for you.

As a society, we should encourage discussions about real problems. The perfect world we often see in the media only represents reality for a few, while many of us deal with hidden challenges and struggles. This book aims to offer different perspectives and remind us that it's okay not to be okay, even in a world where social media makes emotions look flawless.

Emotional abuse isn't always obvious; it can be as subtle as being ignored or lacking affection.

Speak up about it.

Mental health matters!!

ACKNOWLEDGEMENT

Gratitude unfurls its wings as I pen down these words, a heartfelt symphony of appreciation for all those who illuminated my path on this incredible journey.

To my husband, whose unwavering support and unending patience have been the foundation upon which this book was built. Your belief in me and the stories I sought to share was a constant reminder of the power of partnership. Your love and encouragement breathed life into these narratives, and for that, I am endlessly thankful.

To the women whose stories grace these pages, your courage, vulnerability, and resilience have inspired me beyond words. Through your experiences, you have not only enriched this book but have also offered a beacon of strength to others who tread similar paths.

To my family and friends, your encouragement, words of wisdom, and unwavering faith fueled my creative spirit. Your presence in my life has been a constant reminder of the importance of community.

And finally, to the pregnancy journey itself—the highs and lows, the triumphs and challenges. Each step has been a lesson, each moment a revelation. This book is a testament to the beauty of embracing life's intricate tapestry.

Table of Contents

CHAPTER - 1

BREAKING THE CHAINS OF TRADITION

It was 3:30 pm in a middle-class house; the sun's hot rays filtered through the curtains from the adjacent balcony, casting a gentle glow on the pregnant woman diligently working inside the kitchen. The kitchen looked a bit messy, with lots of unwashed utensils around. There were mango peels lying here and there on the slab. A strong odour emanated from the dustbin kept under the sink, making it look like a complete mess.

Sagarika, a woman with determination on her face, balanced her pregnancy and job responsibilities. She gently wiped off a bead of sweat, appearing a bit tired and fully aware that handling both work and household chores simultaneously was challenging. Perhaps, she felt a sense of guilt even though it wasn't her fault. Her movements were cautious, mindful of her delicate state, as she tried to balance her work responsibilities with the growing discomfort within. Amidst the clinking pots and sizzling pans, soft sighs escaped her lips, revealing the struggle she faced in coping with her professional duties and the physical challenges of pregnancy. The warmth of the kitchen seemed to intensify her exhaustion, causing a thin layer of sweat to glisten on her forehead.

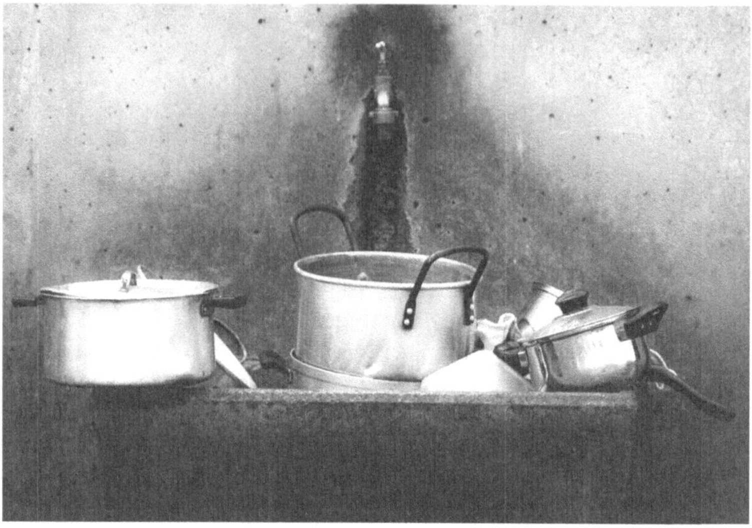

She cleaned the utensils as fast as she could while also glancing at her laptop to respond to the pings she was receiving on Microsoft Teams. Just then, Sagarika's mother-in-law, Mrs. Verma, entered the room with some cut veggies in her basket. She observed Sagarika's chores with a hint of disapproval. "Back in the 1990s, when I was pregnant, I worked hard and managed everything," Mrs. Verma said, her voice tinged with nostalgia and a touch of superiority. Sagarika paused for a moment, her heart sinking as her mind was flooded with mixed emotions. She respected her mother-in-law, but the comparison stung. After all, times had changed, and so had the expectations and pressures on modern women. Societal roles had evolved, and more women, like Sagarika, had embraced both work and personal life with grace and courage. As a first-time pregnant woman, she wasn't aware of the challenges and hardships that would come her way.

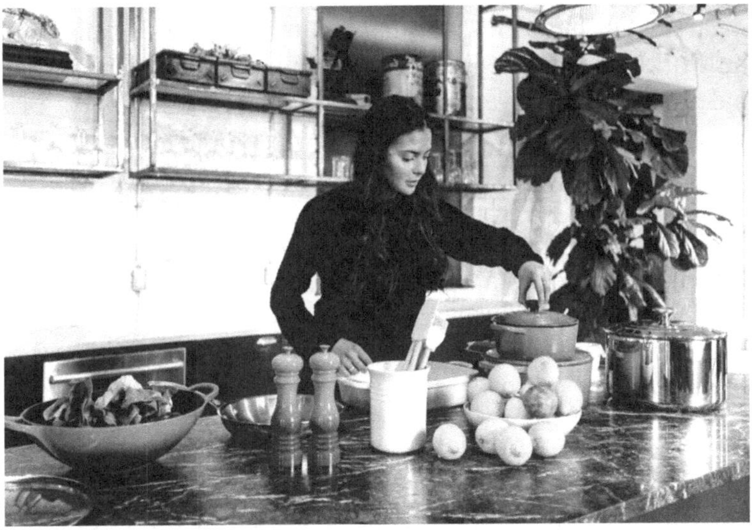

"I know, Ma," Sagarika replied, trying to maintain her composure. "But times have changed, and women today have different responsibilities. Many of us work and support our families financially. It's not that I don't want to help with household chores, but pregnancy has its challenges, and I'm doing my best."

"So, what? I had two pregnancies. I used to go to school to teach and then come back and do all the household chores," replied Mrs. Verma.

"But working at school and coming back by 12, and then working 9 am to 6 pm in today's professional world, where I don't get a single minute off work is different, Ma. Each woman's body is different, and our lifestyles have changed drastically over the years. The food we eat, the environment we live in—everything affects our health. It's not fair to compare the past with the present," Sagarika continued.

Mrs. Verma (Rolling eyes), "Different or not, it's just an excuse. I never had the luxury of remote work, and I still handled everything just fine. I don't understand why you can't manage simple household tasks."

Sagarika felt hurt, "It's not that I can't manage. It's just that the workload is immense, and I sometimes need help or your understanding."

Mrs. Verma, "Help? Why should you need help? In my time, we didn't have all these gadgets and appliances, and we managed fine without any help."

Sagarika replied in a defensive tone, "Technology doesn't always make things easier. It might save time in some aspects, but the expectations and workload have also increased.

I am handling my responsibilities, but I'm also trying to find a balance between work and home. It's not easy, especially when there's little support. Also, there are layoffs going on everywhere."

Mrs. Verma, "You're just not trying hard enough. It's your duty to take care of the house and your husband. Maybe if you focused less on your job, you'd have more time for everything else."

"My job is essential too, and I contribute to this family's well-being. It's not fair to expect me to sacrifice my career entirely just to meet your standards," Sagarika replied.

"Young women these days are so selfish. In my time, we knew our place and didn't question our duties," Mrs. Verma retorted angrily.

Mrs. Verma's expression hardened as she began to disapprove of Sagarika's words. "Is this how you speak to your elders? I didn't say anything wrong. I've told you the reality. In my neighborhood, there's a girl named Richa who wakes up in the morning, cooks food, and then goes to the office. You're wasting half of your money on maids and house helps. I want you to save your money and keep it for your children."

Sagarika repeated, “Times have changed, and women now have more opportunities and choices. I won't apologize for trying to balance both my career and home life.”

Mrs. Verma looked taken aback for a moment, her mind struggling to reconcile old beliefs with the realities of the present. She saw her daughter-in-law's determination, the fire in her eyes, and the burden she carried with grace. Yet, she resisted acknowledging Sagarika's point of view.

“Balance? It's just an excuse for not wanting to put in the effort. If you can't handle it all, maybe you're just not cut out for this role,” Mrs. Verma defended her argument.

“Your judgment and criticism only make things harder for me. I'm doing my best, and I wish you would understand and support me instead of constantly blaming me.”

Mrs. Verma tried to intervene further, “I don’t know what your expectations are. I have never seen anyone in my life complaining about household chores. It is the easiest and quickest thing on earth and it is for your husband's health.” But then Sagarika quickly jumped in.

She understood the manipulation and replied, "But at the cost of my health, Maa? I work for 14 hours in the office just to buy some comfort, don’t I? Moreover, if I earn money, it helps your son survive in the metro city. On top of that, I try my best to ensure that everything is done perfectly, and I myself check everything in the kitchen."

Mrs. Verma went berserk, "I have examples where pregnant ladies work and handle the house as well. You don’t want to take any responsibility at all."

Sagarika fell silent, not wanting to prolong the argument. She thought it was time to let go of outdated norms and embrace the changing world around her.

In the silence that followed, Sagarika's thoughts expanded to a larger perspective. It wasn't just about her and her mother-in-law; it was about the generations to come. She contemplated the weight of traditional expectations that had been passed down through the years, even though they no longer aligned with modern reality. Sagarika's heart ached for a world where women were burdened by societal and family expectations, and their worth was measured by how well they adhered to outdated norms. With newfound determination, Sagarika decided to confront the situation directly. She understood it wasn't just about her mother-in-law; it was about challenging societal attitudes toward women. That evening, she gathered her courage and shared her thoughts with her husband, Raj. It was a gloomy evening and Sagarika greeted Raj as he arrived home from the office. He went to the balcony for fresh air. The balcony was adorned with wall grass and floor grass. In front of him stood an image of a large Buddha fountain, surrounded by plant pots. A small coffee table sat in the middle, with two chairs on each side. From the 12th floor, he could observe children playing in the society park.

While lost in thought, he was interrupted by a faint, feeble sound.

"How was your day at the office?" Sagarika asked politely.

"Yeah, it was good, just a bit tiring TBH."

"I wanted to talk to you about something," Sagarika said, gazing out at the balcony.

"You seem a bit upset. Is everything alright with your health?" Raj was growing nervous.

Sagarika proceeded to share everything that had been happening over the past few weeks.

Raj listened intently as Sagarika expressed her feelings about the expectations placed upon her, not just during her pregnancy but in all aspects of her life.

"I think your mother's expectations are far too much for me. I'm struggling at the office as well. I feel overwhelmed. I have to work 14 hours every day, and Mom was saying she worked while at school. Why should we even compare? Back then, she didn't have any complications, right? Unlike me dealing with subchorionic hematoma."

Raj responded, "Don't let her words bother you. She loves you but doesn't know how to express it. She's had a life where she managed both. That's probably why she has these expectations."

"What? So, I'm not managing both? In her time, she probably taught for 2 hours and took a 5-hour break. She used to come back home at 1 and rest peacefully. She had a joint family to take care of cooking and household chores. Plus, she had good health, and her babies were born when she was 19. I'm 27 and already dealing with complications," Sagarika replied.

Raj understood the weight Sagarika carried, and they had a heartfelt conversation about breaking free from these traditional chains. However, Sagarika found herself disappointed once again when Raj hesitated to confront his mother's judgmental behavior. He tried to pacify her instead of directly addressing the issue and offering support.

In the following weeks, Sagarika's discussions with Raj and her mother-in-law didn't lead to the desired change. Mrs. Verma remained stubborn, criticizing Sagarika's choices and dismissing her concerns. This constant belittling took a toll on Sagarika emotionally, adding to the physical challenges of pregnancy. She felt increasingly isolated and longed for the support she desperately needed during this vulnerable time. The weight of unrealistic expectations started affecting her mental well-being.

One evening, after yet another confrontation with her mother-in-law, Sagarika broke down in tears. Hormonal changes combined with the lack of electricity in the society had made the night particularly difficult. She hadn't been able to sleep due to the non-functioning AC. When she woke up, she was drenched in sweat and completely drained of energy. She contemplated taking a day off from work, prepared her cup of tea, and went back to bed.

Her house help arrived and prepared breakfast for Raj. Raj, already late for work, rushed down the stairs to catch his cab.

"She'll probably sleep until 10 am and then talk about how active she is," Mrs. Verma commented to the house help, Sunita.

Sunita, who lacked context, agreed, "Yes, these days, ladies don't seem to realize the importance of staying active during pregnancy."

Overhearing this conversation, Sagarika was infuriated. She felt suffocated by the constant judgment and comparison, yearning for someone to empathize with her struggles and provide the emotional support she craved. She went to the kitchen and said, "Do you ever see that I work for 14 hours? Do you understand how painful that is?"

"Why do you always undermine the work I do for the office? Isn't that important too?"

Mrs. Verma responded, "You don't know how to balance both aspects, and it's causing problems. You always prioritize your office. In fact, you can't even step into the kitchen to see what's being cooked for Raj."

"But why should I? Isn't that what I pay Sunita for?" retorted Sagarika.

"That's your problem. You'll never realize your mistakes," Mrs. Verma remarked.

Feeling overwhelmed and desperate for solace, Sagarika confided in her close friend, Rhea. Rhea listened attentively, her heart going out to Sagarika as she recounted her painful experiences. Rhea offered a shoulder to lean on and reassured Sagarika that she wasn't alone in her feelings.

"Sagarika, it's okay to feel this way. Pregnancy can be challenging, both physically and emotionally. You deserve kindness, understanding, and respect, especially during this time," Rhea gently said.

Rhea's words deeply resonated with Sagarika, and for the first time in weeks, she felt a glimmer of hope. She realized she didn't have to accept the unfair treatment from her mother-in-law. She could set boundaries, prioritize her well-being, and the well-being of her unborn child.

Summoning courage, Sagarika faced her mother-in-law, took a deep breath, and spoke from her heart. "Maa, I understand you have your beliefs and expectations, but I need you to see things from my perspective too. Pregnancy is challenging for me, and I need your support and empathy. Comparing me to others or the past only adds unnecessary pressure and stress. I'm doing my best, and I hope you can respect my choices and decisions."

Mrs. Verma initially appeared taken aback by Sagarika's assertiveness, but something in her daughter-in-law's eyes pierced through the walls of judgment.

"I only wanted what I thought was best for you, but I see now that my attempts have driven a wedge between us."

Certainly, the author can depict Mrs. Verma as a traditional and unyielding character who clings to her orthodox beliefs.

As weeks turned into months, Sagarika found herself facing increasing challenges with her mother-in-law, Mrs. Verma. Despite Sagarika's efforts to explain her modern perspective and changing societal roles, Mrs. Verma remained staunchly traditional and unwavering in her beliefs.

Mrs. Verma continued to pressure Sagarika to follow her example, adhere to traditional customs, and prioritize household duties over her career. She firmly believed that a woman's primary role was to be a homemaker and a devoted wife, particularly during pregnancy and after childbirth. This clash of values generated tension and friction in their relationship.

One evening, during a family dinner, Mrs. Verma remarked, "Sagarika, you should focus more on household chores and prepare for the baby's arrival. It's not appropriate for you to be so engrossed in your work while carrying a child. In our time, women knew their place and didn't neglect their responsibilities."

Sagarika took a deep breath, struggling to remain composed. She responded, "I understand where you're coming from, maa, but times have changed. Many women, including myself, balance both work and family responsibilities. Having a fulfilling career is important for me, and it also supports our family."

Mrs. Verma shook her head, unconvinced. "This modern lifestyle might suit some, but it's not suitable for a woman about to become a mother. I worry about my grandchild's well-being. You should focus on being a good mother and wife, not chasing after career ambitions."

An uncomfortable silence filled the room as both women held onto their beliefs, unwilling to yield. Sagarika felt frustrated and disheartened by Mrs. Verma's lack of understanding and refusal to acknowledge the validity of her choices.

Caught between respecting her mother-in-law and staying true to her own beliefs, Sagarika attempted to find a middle ground. She participated in some rituals out of respect for family traditions but also asserted her need for personal space and choices during pregnancy.

However, clashes between Mrs. Verma's orthodox beliefs and Sagarika's modern outlook persisted, straining their relationship. Sagarika increasingly felt isolated and unsupported during a period when she needed understanding and love the most.

One day, as Sagarika seeks comfort in her husband, Raj, she expresses her frustrations. "Raj, I respect your mother, but her constant insistence on following outdated customs and disregarding my choices is affecting me deeply. I want her to understand that times have changed, and I have the right to make my own decisions."

Raj listens to Sagarika empathetically but feels torn between his wife and his mother. He loves and respects both of them, struggling to bridge the gap between their differing beliefs.

Finally, Raj confronts his mother about the impact of her actions on Sagarika. "Ma, I understand that you want the best for Sagarika and our baby, but your insistence on traditional practices is causing her stress and anxiety. We need to support her choices and respect her beliefs, just as she respects ours."

Mrs. Verma's initial reaction is defensive; she dismisses Raj's concerns, asserting that her ways are the only right ways. However, deep down, she realizes that her rigid beliefs might be pushing her son away.

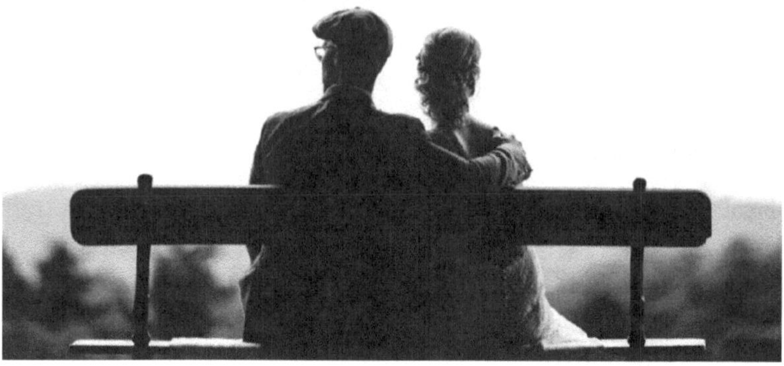

The author notes that such orthodox beliefs, which emphasize balancing both work and home responsibilities, can potentially cause stress for pregnant women due to a variety of reasons. It's important to recognize that these beliefs can vary widely depending on cultural, religious, and societal norms. However, some common themes contribute to stress during pregnancy:

Expectations of Perfection: These beliefs uphold traditional gender roles, pressuring pregnant women to excel both in their careers and as homemakers. Striving for perfection in both areas can become overwhelming and lead to stress.

Lack of Support: Balancing work and home responsibilities becomes more challenging during pregnancy due to physical and emotional changes. When such beliefs discourage seeking help or support, pregnant women might feel isolated and unable to ask for assistance.

Limited Flexibility: Some orthodox beliefs might discourage flexible work arrangements or adjustments for pregnant women. This inflexibility can lead to stress as women struggle to manage work demands alongside their health and preparations for childbirth.

Guilt and Self-Blame: The expectation to excel in both work and home roles can result in feelings of guilt and self-blame if pregnant women believe they are not meeting these expectations. This emotional burden can heighten stress levels.

Health Concerns: Pregnancy brings its own set of physical and emotional challenges. Orthodox beliefs that prioritize work and home responsibilities might not allow for adequate rest and self-care during pregnancy, potentially causing health issues and increased stress.

Cultural Stigma: In certain orthodox societies, there might be a stigma associated with prioritizing personal needs over family and work duties. Pregnant women may fear judgment or ostracization if they express the need to reduce their workload or take time off.

Lack of Empowerment: If these beliefs discourage women from advocating for their needs or asserting boundaries, pregnant women might feel disempowered to make decisions that prioritize their health and well-being.

Uncertain Work Situation: If these beliefs discourage women from openly discussing their pregnancy or maternity leave plans, pregnant women might worry about potential negative impacts on their careers, leading to stress and anxiety.

To mitigate the stress caused by these orthodox beliefs, fostering **open communication** within families, communities, and workplaces is crucial. **Encouraging support** networks and providing flexible work arrangements can significantly alleviate the stress pregnant women experience. Additionally, **promoting education and awareness** about the physical and emotional challenges of pregnancy can help challenge traditional beliefs and encourage a more balanced and healthy approach to pregnancy and work-life balance.

In the end, Sagarika's story isn't about triumphing over Mrs. Verma's orthodox beliefs, but about finding common ground and building a bridge of understanding between two generations. It's a tale of growth, compassion, and the power of love to break down barriers and bring people closer together.

Here are some examples of how pregnant women might feel and express themselves in any community. These sentences are translated into English while maintaining their original intent.

"Absolutely. The in-laws have devised ways of assigning tasks so that the daughter-in-law doesn't get any rest".

"The way it was before the daughter-in-law came, it could continue afterward as well. Honestly, in times like these, women tend to become each other's enemies. I feel that if you can't offer help, at least don't subject her to torture".

"Well, in this matter, I think most mother-in-law's way of thinking won't change, whether now or in the future. They tend to expect their daughter-in-law to handle all the work, no matter how it's done. And when it's time for the baby to be born, they'll remind her of all those things they did. "I did this, I did that, and everything turned out fine".

"I often reply back saying that when you did those things, the times were different. Today's era is not the same as the earlier times when traditions like wearing a veil, dressing in saris, and staying confined were prevalent. So, please don't bring up those old-time customs".

"MIL should stay normal instead of forcing the heart to do something for the sake of work. This mother-in-law doesn't impart this wisdom even to her own daughter".

CHAPTER 2

UNSEEN STRUGGLES AT OFFICE

The office buzzed with activity as the clock struck 6 pm, marking the end of yet another busy workday. Colleagues hurriedly gathered their belongings, exchanging quick goodbyes as they prepared to leave before the impending rainstorm outside. In the midst of this bustling scene, Samiksha Tiwari, a five-month pregnant woman, navigated through the crowd with visible weariness. She was dressed in a loose yellow co-ord outfit adorned with a flowery pattern all over. The pregnancy had added a glow to her face, making her look even prettier than usual. However, fatigue was evident on her face, and her hair, once neatly tied in a bun, had become disheveled. Her eyes appeared slightly swollen behind her black spectacles.

Kanika Mantry, Samiksha's boss, who was wearing a salwar kurti, exuded the demeanor of a typical boss. With her fair complexion and moderate height, she wore a white watch on her left wrist that she frequently checked. This continuous watch-checking seemed aimed at making the employees leaving early uncomfortable.

She watched Samiksha's preparations to leave with a discerning eye. A hint of annoyance gnawed at Kanika as she noticed Samiksha getting ready to depart earlier than her colleagues. In Kanika's perspective, it seemed like Samiksha was using her pregnancy as an excuse to leave work early.

Approaching Samiksha with an air of casualness, Kanika remarked, "Heading home early, Samiksha?" Her tone carried a subtle hint of sarcasm.

Samiksha took a deep breath, composing herself. She knew she needed to stand her ground and not let Kanika's comment affect her.

"Yes, Kanika," she replied calmly, "the weather forecast predicts heavy rain, and I don't want to take any chances with my commute."

Nodding, Kanika continued, using the opportunity to make her point indirectly.

"I understand," she said, "but when I was pregnant last year, I worked right up until my delivery. It wasn't easy, but I managed to balance my responsibilities."

The remark struck a chord within Samiksha. While she admired Kanika's dedication, the comparison felt unjust and hurtful. She understood that each pregnancy was unique, and her situation was complicated by placenta previa. Despite her efforts to maintain a positive outlook, Kanika's comment stirred up feelings of frustration and vulnerability.

Deep down, Samiksha recognized the significance of her work and the value she brought to the office. However, she also understood that her body required special care during this critical time. Placenta previa demanded extra caution and attention, and she couldn't disregard her doctor's advice simply to conform to workplace norms.

"So, Kanika, every pregnancy is different, and each body responds uniquely. I'm glad that God didn't give you any pregnancy complications, enabling you to work until your last day," retorted Samiksha.

"I'd also like to remind you that you could work until the end not solely due to your hard work but because you were blessed with a complication-free pregnancy. I deeply admire those who work during pregnancy, and even without complications, giving 100% at work requires significant effort. That's why I used to respect you. Now, think about a woman who is already pregnant and dealing with additional complications," Samiksha added. "Despite all my complications, I gave my all in Q2," Samiksha elaborated.

Amidst the feeling of being misunderstood, Samiksha found a sense of determination growing within her. She realized she didn't need to justify her actions to others or feel guilty about prioritizing her health. The workplace should be a space that supports employees' well-being without subjecting them to unnecessary comparisons or judgments.

Not every office is the same; some places are compassionate, while others discriminate. Pregnant women are put at a disadvantage, and their leaves are treated as excuses.

Even after presenting all her points, Samiksha was met with a very rude response from Kanika.

"See, I agree that you gave your 100%, but taking frequent leaves and leaving the office early may cast you in a negative light, Samiksha. Then, I won't be able to help you anymore. Also, the performance review is just around the corner," retorted Kanika.

Samiksha understood that Kanika was indirectly implying that her ratings might be lowered in the review. However, she didn't prolong the argument and provided a concluding statement.

"I understand that you've been a mother too, but during your time, it was Covid work-from-home period. Hence, you might not fully grasp my struggles at this point. Furthermore, I'm not seeking sympathy from anyone. My work will speak for itself, and I'm not afraid of the appraisal. God has already blessed me with a baby, and I'm confident in the output I've delivered to the organization."

Samiksha also attempted to highlight how her colleagues, including Kanika, wasted around 2 hours every day in the cafeteria/canteen and then pretended to leave late.

She said, "I don't waste my time in the canteen for 3 hours and then extend my day for 3 hours just to gain attention. I believe that if my efficiency is higher and I can complete my work ahead of time, I should help save the company's resources, like internet and electricity costs."

Kanika perceived this as a direct sarcasm and responded, "You don't need to worry about the company's fixed costs too much. If you can work on this marketing campaign and finish it in 2 days, it will significantly reduce acquisition costs and compensate for all fixed costs, won't it?"

Samiksha replied, "Yes, by leaving early, I've already saved the company more than double the cost of this campaign itself. I have the numbers ready to extend this conversation further. However, I'd rather not continue this discussion because if the marketing campaign is going live in 2 days, I should be at my desk working, rather than discussing the company's profit and loss."

Kanika was taken aback by the directness of Samiksha's responses, and she shifted into a vindictive mode.

Samiksha's growing belly made sitting for extended periods uncomfortable, and she frequently needed breaks to stretch her legs. Additionally, she struggled to eat lunch at the appropriate time, with cold chapatis making her meals difficult. Not being able to consume fresh juices on time due to spoilage was another challenge. She often thought about how much easier it was for other women who could work from home.

The washroom was a shared facility, which put Samiksha at a higher risk of developing a UTI. Unfortunately, it wasn't being cleaned properly, and with 45 female staff members on the floor using it, kept it in a messy state.

Samiksha attempted to reach out to her friend Manisha, who had the privilege of working from home, to understand how much easier it was for her.

One evening, Samiksha called Manisha. "Hey, Manisha, you must feel blessed to have the option to work from home during your pregnancy. How do you find it? I ask because I'm really tired from going to the office and struggling to eat properly and on time."

Manisha replied, "Samiksha, the grass always seems greener on the other side. I won't say that working from home is more challenging than going to the office, but it does come with its own set of difficulties. You don't have a fixed time to close your office. There's no routine; you might wake up at 9 am and be in a meeting at 9:30 am. Hormonal changes make you feel isolated, and not seeing anyone all day can lead to increased feelings of depression. Sometimes there's not even time for a bathroom break due to back-to-back calls. Additionally, in a work-from-home setup, every minor issue seems to require a meeting, causing more discussions than necessary. Work-from-home employees often end up sitting for longer hours, leading to various health issues. While we change positions frequently to avoid discomfort, this also leads to back problems. And yes, we may have a personal washroom, but how can we use it if we're in the middle of a meeting? These days, women are conceiving at a later age, around 30 or 31, which means they're often already in mid-management roles and can't put their work at risk. Moreover, when you're in the office, you can lock your home worries away for 8 hours. But for work-from-home employees, home responsibilities like cleaning and spending time with in-laws can easily fall on our shoulders."

Samiksha felt overwhelmed. "You're absolutely right. Every situation comes with its own challenges, and we need to learn how to adapt without constantly comparing ourselves to others."

Manisha added, "That's a valuable lesson for every pregnant woman – never compare your body, baby, and situation with anyone else's."

Meanwhile, Kanika, who had clashed with Samiksha earlier, tried to take advantage of the situation. She approached Sachet, her boss, with a plan to remove Samiksha from a project due to her pregnancy. Kanika believed that Samiksha might not be able to contribute effectively.

Sachet, an IITian married to a successful woman in HR, responded differently. "I may not fully understand this as a man, but pregnancy is not an illness. It comes with its own struggles and challenges. Some women may not be able to contribute as much, but they push themselves harder due to guilt. In this case, we shouldn't remove Samiksha from the project. Instead, let's provide her with flexible hours so she can contribute comfortably and deliver results. Let's avoid making sarcastic comments and refrain from putting her at any disadvantage during pregnancy – that's unethical and illegal."

Kanika's shrewd nature seemed to be overpowering her compassion.

Unaware of the conversation between Kanika and Sachet, Samiksha was deeply concerned about her performance appraisal. As she headed home, she wished for a more compassionate and accommodating work environment. She hoped for a workplace that recognized the unique needs of its employees, especially those facing health challenges during pregnancy. Her wish was for a place that valued not only dedication to work but also understood the significance of self-care and empathy.

The next day, Samiksha decided to take action. She approached Kanika, not confrontationally, but with the intention of initiating a conversation about better support for pregnant employees. She shared her experiences and the challenges she faced due to placenta previa, aiming to raise awareness about the importance of workplace empathy.

However, Kanika dismissed Samiksha's concerns, labelling them as mere excuses. She seemed resistant to understanding the difficulties pregnant women encounter and remained firm in her belief that work commitment should always come first.

On another day, Samiksha was called into Kanika's office, possibly to discuss Q3 guidelines.

"We have Q3 priorities coming up, and there's much to do. You need to prepare," Kanika said.

Samiksha responded, "Kanika, I've sensed a certain unease about my pregnancy and work commitments. I want to assure you that I'm fully dedicated to my role, but I also need some understanding during this crucial time."

"I do appreciate your commitment, but we all have responsibilities. Pregnancy doesn't mean you can't fulfill your professional duties," Kanika retorted.

"I'm not seeking special treatment, Kanika. Just a bit of empathy and flexibility given the circumstances," Samiksha explained.

"I'll try to be understanding, but I hope it won't affect the team's productivity," Kanika said.

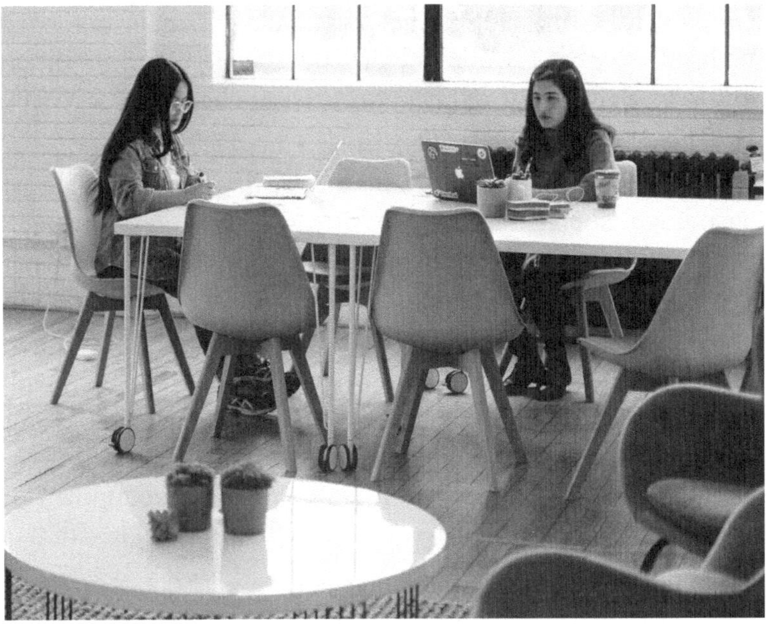

Creating a non-supportive office environment can significantly impact the mental well-being of anyone, including pregnant women. Pregnancy is a sensitive period in a woman's life, and the stress and anxiety caused by an unsupportive workplace can be particularly detrimental. Here are some ways in which a non-supportive office can negatively affect the mental peace of pregnant women:

Lack of Flexibility: If the office doesn't provide flexible work hours or remote work options, pregnant women might struggle with commuting, fatigue, and medical appointments. This lack of flexibility can lead to increased stress and discomfort.

Insensitive Attitudes: Colleagues or supervisors who make insensitive comments about pregnancy, body changes, or maternity leave can create a hostile environment. This can lead to feelings of isolation, anxiety, and even depression.

Unrealistic Workload: If the pregnant woman is burdened with an excessive workload that doesn't take her condition into consideration, it can lead to burnout, stress, and a feeling of being overwhelmed.

Lack of Social Support: If the office culture doesn't encourage social interactions or team bonding, pregnant women might feel excluded or disconnected from their colleagues. This isolation can contribute to feelings of loneliness and anxiety.

Discrimination and Stereotyping: Discrimination based on pregnancy, such as being passed over for promotions or important projects, can damage self-esteem and trigger anxiety. Stereotyping pregnant women as less committed or productive can also negatively impact their mental health.

The author points out that it is not only about Samiksha; there are many employees in India who face insensitive attitudes, unrealistic workloads, and discrimination because of their pregnancy. On top of that, no one realizes the complications because, for many people, "Pregnancy is a normal phase, what's the big deal?"

The author conducted a survey among pregnant women and discovered some of the most hurtful comments received:

- "Wow, you're really getting big! Are you sure there's only one in there?"
- "You must be so hormonal right now. I wouldn't want to be around you."
- "Pregnancy brain strikes again, huh?"
- "Are you planning on coming back to work after the baby? It's so hard to balance both, you know."
- "You're taking a lot of breaks lately. Must be nice to have an excuse to slack off."

- "Your maternity leave is like a vacation! I wish I could take that much time off."
- "Are you sure you're up for this project? I mean, with the baby coming and all."
- "You're still here? I thought you'd be on maternity leave by now."
- "Pregnancy must be the perfect excuse to eat whatever you want, right?"

Pregnant women can seek justice from the court if they face any discrimination like the above. Yes, there have been cases in the past where individuals have filed cases against employers for pregnancy-related discrimination in India. Here are a few examples:

Meera Santosh Pal v. Union of India: In 2016, Meera Santosh Pal, an employee of the Indian Railways, filed a petition alleging that she was denied maternity leave and subjected to discrimination due to her pregnancy. The Bombay High Court ruled in her favor and directed the Railways to ensure compliance with maternity benefits and provide appropriate relief.

Rupa Ashok Hurra v. Ashok Hurra and Anr: This case, although not specifically about pregnancy discrimination, is relevant. In 2002, the Supreme Court of India held that a woman cannot be discriminated against in matters of promotion or seniority on the grounds of her pregnancy or maternity leave. The court upheld the principle of gender equality and non-discrimination.

Nalini S. v. Indian Overseas Bank & Ors: In this case, an employee alleged that her promotion was denied because of her pregnancy. The Madras High Court ordered the bank to reconsider her promotion and ensure that maternity-related leave was not held against her in promotions.

Please note that these examples are not exhaustive and may not cover all the nuances of each case. Laws and regulations evolve, and outcomes can vary based on individual circumstances and interpretations of the law. If you're looking for more detailed information about specific cases, consulting legal databases, news sources, or seeking advice from legal experts familiar with Indian labor laws would be advisable.

It's important for employers to recognize the needs of pregnant employees and create a supportive environment. Providing flexible work options, reasonable accommodations, education for colleagues about sensitivity, clear communication, and fair policies can go a long way in ensuring the mental well-being of pregnant women in the workplace. If you or someone you know is facing challenges in a non-supportive office environment, consider seeking guidance from human resources or support groups for pregnant women.

CHAPTER 3

EMBRACING THE JOURNEY TOGETHER

The office hummed with activity as Divya wrapped up her work for the day. She was seven months pregnant, and as she bid farewell to her colleagues, her thoughts drifted to the one person she longed to see the most – her husband, Rohan. Rohan worked as a Senior Consultant at one of the Big Fours and often had very little time to spend with Divya. He left for the office at 8 am and returned at 10 pm. By then, he was extremely tired to engage in any discussion with Divya. This was due to physical exhaustion and mental preoccupation.

Divya, who was of short stature, extremely fair, and had long hair that reached her knees, felt that this was an important day for her as she was leaving her office for the next six months. She was a little nervous, somewhat happy, and apprehensive about the future. The monsoon in Mumbai had made the weather gloomy, adding to her stress. Her eyes welled up, and the strong winds were playing havoc with her long hair. She walked out onto a gallery to reach the elevator, and her kurti and dupatta swayed in the wind. Her eyes welled up, and her voice was slightly choked as she pressed the "G" button in the lift. Stepping out of the office building, she felt a mix of emotions. Pregnancy had brought immense joy, but it also came with its challenges. While Rohan had taken on the responsibility of providing for the family financially, Divya felt an overwhelming need for something more – emotional support and companionship, someone who could understand the pain behind her seemingly fake smile.

Her heart filled with anticipation as she thought of seeing Rohan waiting for her at home. She imagined him greeting her with a warm smile, eager to listen to her day, and share in her feelings and experiences. She craved his understanding and presence during this significant phase of their lives.

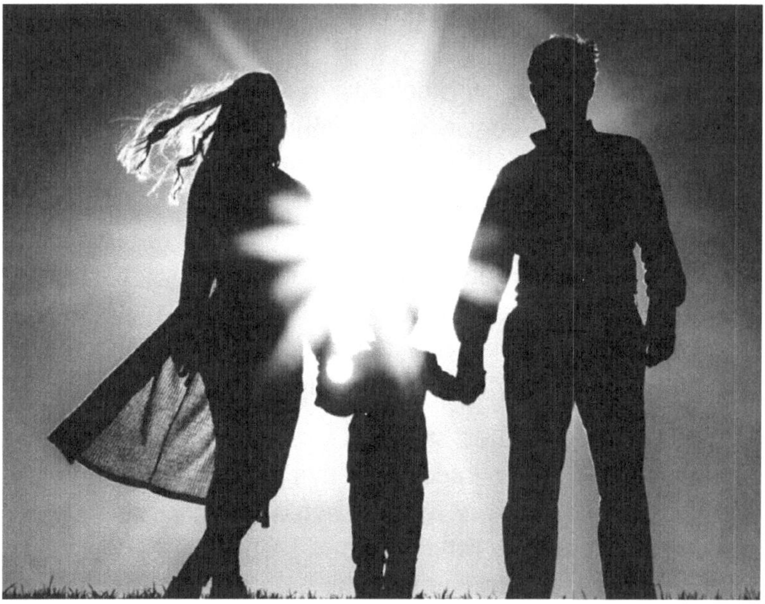

However, reality often fell short of expectations, and Divya found herself grappling with a sense of disappointment. Despite Rohan's good intentions, he often seemed preoccupied with work and other commitments, leaving Divya feeling like she was facing her pregnancy journey alone. She yearned for a deeper connection, someone to lean on when the weight of pregnancy seemed too much to bear.

That day, too, Rohan arrived around 10 pm, and Divya opened the door and greeted him with a smile.

"It was a really tiring day at my office. Kannan told me to come up with the presentation tomorrow morning at 11 am. How is that possible on earth? I am overloaded with work after the layoffs and team size reduction. Anyways, how was your day, Divya?" asked Rohan.

After listening to Rohan's stress, she simply said, "Yes, it was fine," replied Divya.

Divya had a lot to tell him, like her upcoming leave and how suffocating she felt. She wanted to share about the indifference she sensed in her boss's eyes as she bid farewell to the office. She thought maybe this office wouldn't need her after her maternity leave. She even contemplated updating her resume to apply elsewhere. However, she didn't tell Rohan anything and remained silent. Often, when one can't express their feelings, they become mentally burdened. This was happening with Divya.

As days turned into weeks, Divya found herself needing more than just physical comfort. She needed someone who could empathize with her emotional struggles and be a pillar of strength in moments of vulnerability. The challenges of pregnancy were not just physical; they took a toll on her mental well-being as well.

One evening, as the sun began its descent, Divya and Rohan sat together in the living room. Their spacious living room had a TV cabinet placed in the center of one wall. To the left of the TV was a guest bedroom, and to the right, the kitchen. Their bedroom was right next to the sofa, and a second guest room was on the left side of the sofa. The interior design gave the room a polished and classy look, making it seem well-decorated.

While the room was bathed in a warm, golden glow, Divya's heart felt heavy. She knew she had to share her feelings with Rohan; she couldn't keep them bottled up any longer.

"Rohan," she began, her voice soft but resolute, "I need to talk to you about something that's been bothering me." Rohan turned toward her, concern in his eyes, and nodded for her to continue.

"I know you're doing your best to take care of me financially," Divya started, "and I appreciate that. But what I really need right now is your emotional support. I feel so lonely at times, overwhelmed by everything that's happening. I want to share my thoughts and feelings with you, to feel like we're in this together."

Rohan listened attentively as Divya poured her heart out. She explained the challenges she faced as her body changed, the restrictions on her activities, and the rollercoaster of emotions she experienced daily. She longed for a deeper connection with Rohan, one that went beyond mere pleasantries and casual conversation.

"I need you to be there for me, Rohan," she implored, tears welling up in her eyes. "I want us to be partners in this journey, to understand and support each other through all the ups and downs."

Rohan reached out to hold her hand, his expression softening with understanding. "I'm sorry, Divya," he said gently. "I didn't realize how much you were going through. I promise I'll be more present for you. Let's go through this together, as a team."

But was it all true? Divya sensed a disconnect but decided to give it time.

In the days that followed, Rohan made a conscious effort to be more attentive to Divya's needs. He would sit with her during meals, even if it was just for a few minutes, asking about her day and listening to her thoughts. He took time to learn about the changes her body was going through, attending prenatal classes with her and researching ways to provide additional support.

One afternoon, Divya mentioned to Rohan how she felt a bit bored staying at home all day. She hoped he would suggest a small outing or plan a surprise to lift her spirits. However, Rohan's response left her disheartened.

"Who likes going out, Divya?" he said with a sigh. "It's a pain for me to go out after a long day at work. Besides, you're lucky to be working from home and staying here. You have everything you need. I have to work even on weekends. You have the whole day with you, why can't you do something creative?"

Divya was taken aback. She had expected Rohan to understand her need for a change of scenery, a break from the monotony of home life. She had hoped he would empathize and perhaps plan a small dinner out, just the two of them. Instead, she felt like her feelings were dismissed once again. As the weeks passed, Divya struggled with feelings of isolation and sadness. She found herself yearning for the emotional support she craved, and Rohan's lack of understanding left her feeling more alone than ever. She decided to speak to him again.

Divya: sighs "Rohan, I've been feeling really overwhelmed lately. My emotions are all over the place, and I just need your support."

"What do you mean, Divya? You seem fine to me. Is something bothering you? You are not the first pregnant woman in the world. Everyone goes through this, and how can you be so sensitive every time?", asked Rohan.

"It's just that pregnancy hormones are making me feel really sensitive and emotional. I might cry over little things or get upset without any specific reason. It's not something I can control", replied Divya.

"But I've seen you handle stress and emotions before. This can't be that different, right?" Rohan questioned.

"It's not about handling stress, Rohan. These hormonal changes are beyond my control. It's like a roller coaster of feelings. I need you to understand and be patient with me," cried Divya.

"I'm trying to understand, Divya, but it's hard for me to grasp. I mean, I can't relate to what you're going through," replied Rohan.

"I know you can't directly relate, but that's not the point. The point is that I need your empathy and support. When I'm feeling down or upset, I need you to be there for me, even if you don't fully understand," told Divya.

"Sorry, I don't understand. What am I doing wrong? What do I need to do?" asked Rohan in utter disgrace.

"Just be patient and understanding. If I'm feeling down, give me a hug or offer some words of reassurance. It's not about solving the problem but about being there for me," said Divya.

"This pregnancy has become too much of a drama for me to be honest. I mean, I see a lot of women in my office; they seem pretty normal without being this kind of attention seeker. They work in the office and manage both the worlds easily," told Rohan.

"But why can't we **normalize feeling 'NOT OKAY' in pregnancy**? I understand a certain segment of women are courageous and a certain segment are not. I am one of them maybe. Why do you need to compare me with anyone else? I am not lying, and whatever I feel, I can only confide in my partner, right?" Divya responded tearfully.

She rushed to her right, where her bedroom was, and locked the door from inside and slept. Rohan didn't even come to talk to her, and he slept in another room, citing a headache.

Fast forward to 3 days later…

A close friend of Divya's, Neha, came over to visit. Neha had recently become a mother and understood the challenges of pregnancy and early motherhood firsthand. She could sense the emotional toll it was taking on Divya and decided to have a heart-to-heart conversation with her.

"Divya," Neha began gently,

"I know it's not easy, and it's okay to feel overwhelmed. But have you tried talking to Rohan about how you feel?"

"I did," Divya replied, her voice tinged with sadness. "But it seems like he doesn't fully understand or take my feelings seriously."

Neha nodded empathetically. "Sometimes, people need time to understand and adjust. You've got to keep communicating with him, let him know how you feel and what you need."

Divya took Neha's advice to heart. That evening, she sat down with Rohan once again on the balcony, offering a bowl of snacks to him. This time, she approached the conversation with patience and understanding. She reiterated her feelings and emphasized the significance of his presence in her life.

"I need you, Rohan," she said, her voice steady but full of emotion. "I don't just want you to be here physically; I need your emotional support, your companionship. Pregnancy is not just about the physical aspects; it's about the emotional journey we take together."

There are a lot of households these days where husbands take care of wives in pregnancy by being a financial support but fail to understand her emotionally. A lady goes through a lot mentally and physically, and she needs a lot of motivation and encouragement. Being there for each other doesn't mean being physically present, but it means being psychologically connected to each other.

The author says, the one person a woman can confide her feelings with is her husband, and all husbands need to be more supportive. Just think, where we are heading as a society? If we can't keep the mother of our child happy, what is the purpose of living? Why do we let mothers suffer with pain, emotional toll, and everything? We should also adjust a little bit. She is adjusting physically, her body is bigger than ever, her face is swollen, her baby bump not letting her sleep. When someone next to you is facing such issues, can we not just sacrifice our sleep and comfort for one day to make her feel supported?

Let's see some of the examples of the comments from Pregnant ladies about their husbands and how overwhelming are they:

"I have no expectations from my husband; my husband doesn't care about me at all, whether it's during pregnancy or not".

"My husband also doesn't seem to have any significance for them (referring to the ladies' parents), everything was fine for the first year of marriage, but now

"Whose husband spends time with you all after delivery? My husband is always engrossed in his

"Hello moms, my husband doesn't pay any attention to me, and neither do my in-laws believe me. I stay with my parents during pregnancy. It is my 8th month and my husband never visit me ever neither asks about my well-being, I feel like a single mother. He doesn't even give me money for personal expenses".

"Please help me. My mother-in-law is saying negative things about me to my husband. What should I do? My husband isn't even talking to me".

"My husband and his mother both nag me all the time. My husband doesn't care about me even a little and just believes her mom. What should I do? Why are MILs like this"?

There are several ways in which a husband can provide support to pregnant women:

Engage with the Baby: Taking time each day to talk to the baby and reassuring his wife that they are in this journey and together can foster a sense of togetherness and connection.

Avoid Body Judgment: Refraining from commenting on weight gain or making any sarcastic remarks is crucial. A sensitive approach towards physical changes is essential.

Provide Motivation: Encouraging words go a long way. Remind her that the challenges she's facing during pregnancy are temporary and that their upcoming baby will bring immense joy to the family.

Handle Mood Swings: Patiently listening during mood swings and responding with empathy rather than reacting can make a significant difference. Extra attention during these moments can provide great comfort.

Act as a Shield: Being a strong presence in front of both his parents and his wife's family, shielding her from unnecessary judgments, and advocating for her needs can create a positive and supportive environment.

Offer Physical Comfort: Providing physical comfort through actions like back rubs, foot massages, or drawing a warm bath can help alleviate any physical discomfort she may be experiencing.

Attend Prenatal Appointments: Being present at prenatal appointments, ultrasounds, and check-ups showcases active involvement and enhances understanding of the pregnancy's progress.

Remember, supporting a pregnant partner not only helps her feel emotionally secure but also strengthens the bond between husband and wife during this transformative phase.

CHAPTER 4

EMPATHY UNVEILED

The scorching sun beat down on the day of the convocation ceremony at Staplewood University. The atmosphere was filled with excitement and anticipation as students prepared to receive their degrees. Among them was Richa, an outstanding student who was four months pregnant and about to be awarded the gold medal for her remarkable academic achievements in her MBA (Master of Business Administration).

Richa's heart swelled with pride as she stood among her fellow graduates, her belly gently cradling the precious life growing within her. However, as the hours dragged on in the unyielding heat, Richa felt her energy wane. She tried to keep a smile on her face, but the dizziness and light bleeding were becoming harder to ignore. She was wearing a white saree with a red blouse and looked even more beautiful than usual because of her pregnancy glow. Tall and fair, she carried with her a bag of impressive academic accolades.

Throughout the ceremony, Richa's friends Sumit and Saurabh were present. However, they were oblivious to the struggle Richa was enduring. Having never witnessed pregnancy complications in their own family, they brushed off any signs of discomfort as mere theatrics.

Sumit, a lean guy from Bihar with a fairly average height, glanced at Richa from time to time. Whenever he asked if she was okay, she assured him that she was fine. She didn't want to burden him or dampen the celebration with her struggles. Saurabh, also from Bihar, resembled an older version of Amitabh Bachchan. Wearing a white shirt with a yellowish stain at the back, he attempted to infuse humor into conversations with Sumit. Richa, Sumit, and Saurabh were seated in the auditorium according to their roll numbers. Since Sumit and Saurabh had consecutive roll numbers, they were seated together, while Richa was in a different place. Richa felt nauseated during the ceremony as her first-trimester nausea hadn't completely subsided. She sipped an ORS tetra pack intermittently to alleviate the discomfort. Additionally, due to some complications, she experienced light bleeding, and the white saree was adding to her discomfort.

As the ceremony progressed, Richa's name was called, and she proudly walked up to the dais to receive her gold medal. The chief guest and her faculty were very proud of Richa's achievements, as they had witnessed her work diligently for every exam, even the small quizzes. The entire auditorium echoed with her name as applause filled the air. However, as is often the case, sometimes friends are the ones who fail to share in your accomplishments. Sumit and Saurabh clapped half-heartedly, their faces masking thinly veiled resentment. When Richa returned to her seat, she overheard Saurabh muttering to Sumit, "She always gets what she wants."

Unaware of the turmoil within Richa's heart, Sumit smirked and replied, "Yeah, she's just good at memorizing things, that's all. That's why she's the medallist."

Richa's heart sank at their callous comments, feeling hurt and betrayed by the lack of empathy from her own friends. She had always believed they would support her, but their indifference and judgment left her feeling isolated and misunderstood.

As the ceremony dragged on, Richa's condition worsened, but she continued to put on a brave front. After the ceremony, Saurabh reached out to Richa to congratulate her.

"Hey, congrats, shall we go and meet Professor Pranav for the pictures?" asked Saurabh.

"No, Saurabh, please go ahead and take your photographs. I may not be able to walk further; I am not feeling well, to be honest," said Richa.

Unfazed by her response, Saurabh shrugged, telling Sumit, "Pregnancy can't be that difficult. She's just being dramatic. My wife delivered a baby last year, and she went to Lonavala in her 4th month of pregnancy. She was perfectly fine, even though she's 4 years older than Richa. Who knows what kind of complications prevent her from even walking to the professor?"

Sumit chimed in, "Yeah, she always makes a big deal out of everything."

Unaware of the silent struggle Richa was facing, they carried on with the celebration, never bothering to check on her well-being or offer any support.

As the day drew to a close, Richa finally managed to escape the crowd and find a quiet spot to rest. She felt a mix of emotions—pride for her achievements and disappointment at the lack of empathy from her best friends. She reflected on how they had never truly understood her, dismissing her feelings and struggles as insignificant. She longed for them to see the reality of her experiences and support her in her journey of motherhood.

Richa called Sumit the next day and said, "Hey, sorry, I was a bit lost that day due to my health. How are you guys doing?"

"Yeah, we are doing good. In fact, we have multiple pictures from the ceremony, and some are even in newspapers. We had a great time. I wish I could also get a medal like you. How did you manage to study during your pregnancy? I mean, someone who can't even walk at convocation, how can that person manage the entire semester?" replied Sumit in a sarcastic tone.

Richa longed for them to understand her pain and be there for her during this vulnerable time, but it seemed that her plea for empathy fell on deaf ears.

"Yeah, Sumit, my pregnancy had a lot of complications in the first trimester. You have always seen normal pregnancies, so maybe you can't relate to me. Honestly, I don't care too much because I feel a lack of empathy is common these days," Richa burst out her frustrations.

"Yes, I have seen complications in pregnancies with my sister, but she used to manage it so gracefully. You were also smiling during the entire convocation, right? How did your health deteriorate all of a sudden when I asked you to come to the professor? I think you were perfectly fine before that, right? Even your medal pictures that have come show you smiling," Sumit added.

Richa sensed a bit of jealousy from Sumit for not receiving the medal and also a lack of compassion towards her pregnancy.

"So, if I smile, doesn't mean I am not in pain. I think this is the basic education that we are given. Also, it is often said,

'Don't judge a book by its cover.' I was in excruciating pain that day, bleeding and tense about the growth of my newborn. I had subchorionic hematoma and was asked to travel with precautions. I still came to college to get my degree in front of my parents, and getting a gold medal was the cherry on top. I had mixed feelings. But I had never thought that I was being constantly monitored by your camera-like eyes," retorted Richa.

"I think this has gone too far. I really don't understand why people use pregnancies as an excuse," replied Sumit.

Richa interjected, "Excuse me, just because you didn't get the medal doesn't mean you can vent your frustration on me. I'm not sure how you managed your wife and sister during pregnancy with such chauvinistic behavior, but may they be blessed in their next life. If you haven't seen complicated pregnancies, it doesn't mean they don't exist. Also, I feel like I'm talking to someone from kindergarten, so let's just leave it at that. Goodbye forever."

She considered calling Saurabh to tell him the whole story, as she had lost one best friend that day. However, she thought they might discuss it together and it could lead to more damage than damage control. So, she decided to distance herself from Saurabh as well.

The author believes that this isn't an isolated incident. Many examples like this exist where pregnancy is treated as an excuse and unwarranted criticism prevails in the modern world. Here are a few examples that illustrate the type of behavior that can be hurtful or unsympathetic towards pregnant women. Please note that these examples are paraphrased to illustrate the insensitive comments or actions directed towards pregnant women that you may or may not have come across online.

1. Unsolicited Parenting Advice:

- "You're going to let your child do that? I wouldn't if I were you. You'll regret it later."

2. Body and Weight Comments:

- "Wow, you've gained so much weight! Are you sure you're not having twins?"

3. Comparisons to Others' Pregnancies:

- "My cousin didn't have any problems during her pregnancy. You must be exaggerating."

4. Jokes About Hormones:

- "Are you sure you're not overreacting because of those pregnancy hormones?"

5. Disregarding Feelings:

- "You're acting like your life is so hard. Wait till you actually have a baby!"

6. Implying Incompetence:

- "You won't be able to handle that project. Pregnancy is already making you so scatter-brained."

7. Criticism of Choices:

- "You're still working out? You should be resting and taking it easy."

8. Minimizing Pain and Discomfort:

- "It can't be that bad. People have been having babies for centuries."

9. Comparing Pregnancies to Illness:

- "You're acting like you're sick all the time. Pregnancy isn't an illness, you know."

10. Body Comments and Comparisons:

- "Your belly is so small compared to other pregnant women I've seen. Is everything okay?"

11. Unwanted Predictions:

- "I bet you're going to be one of those super anxious moms, worrying about everything."

12. Invasive Questions:

- "Are you planning a natural birth? Oh, you should definitely consider it!"

It's important for friends to be mindful of their words and actions, especially when interacting with pregnant women. Offering support, understanding, and positive encouragement can go a long way in making the pregnant woman feel valued and respected during this transformative time in her life.

As Richa's pregnancy progressed, she faced more challenges, both physical and emotional. She endured sleepless nights, morning sickness, and the fear of the unknown. Throughout it all, Sumit and Saurabh remained indifferent, never bothering to inquire about her well-being.

Richa learned to find solace in herself and sought support from friends and online communities of expecting mothers who understood her struggles.

Pregnancy, a beautiful and transformative journey, is not without its challenges. For many expectant mothers, it can be a rollercoaster of emotions, both physically and mentally. However, the experience can be further complicated when those closest to them fail to understand their struggles. Moreover, some women have to face complications that add to their difficulties.

When a pregnant woman feels misunderstood, it can be an incredibly isolating and disheartening experience. She may be grappling with a myriad of emotions, ranging from joy and excitement to anxiety and exhaustion. Yet, when her loved ones dismiss or overlook her feelings, it can leave her feeling unheard and invalidated. A pregnant woman may long for empathy and support, especially from her partner and family. Pregnancy comes with its share of physical discomforts like morning sickness, backaches, and fatigue. Emotionally, she may experience mood swings and heightened sensitivity.

In times of vulnerability, a pregnant woman needs reassurance that her feelings are valid and that she is not alone in her struggles. When she doesn't receive this understanding, it can lead to feelings of frustration, sadness, and even resentment towards those around her. The lack of understanding can also impact her self-esteem and confidence. She may question her own emotions and doubt whether her experiences are being exaggerated or overlooked. The weight of feeling misunderstood may further contribute to her stress and anxiety, potentially affecting her overall well-being and the well-being of the unborn child.

Often, pregnant women may try to put on a brave face, not wanting to burden others with their worries. They may smile through the discomfort, minimizing their struggles to protect their loved ones from worry or stress. However, this can lead to a cycle of silence and suppression, preventing the pregnant woman from seeking the support and understanding she desperately needs.

It's crucial for everyone, especially those close to a pregnant woman, to be attuned to her needs and emotions. Offering a compassionate ear and a helping hand can make a world of difference in her journey. As society evolves, it is essential to break away from traditional gender roles and expectations and to promote a culture of empathy and support for pregnant women. Recognizing the unseen struggles of expectant mothers and fostering an environment of understanding can lead to more fulfilling and empowering pregnancy experiences.

The author says that the journey of pregnancy is one that deserves utmost care, empathy, and understanding. Being there for a pregnant woman, truly hearing her experiences, and offering unwavering support can make a significant impact on her well-being and create a positive and memorable pregnancy journey for both her and her loved ones.

CHAPTER 5

THE DUALITY OF PREGNANCY ON SOCIAL MEDIA

In the age of social media, pregnancy has taken on a new and glamorous facade. Influencers and celebrities flood our feeds with pictures of their carefree pregnancies, seemingly unaffected by any challenges. They portray an image of women who effortlessly juggle glamorous lifestyles and motherhood, leaving many to wonder if they, too, should be living the same picture-perfect experience.

The author admires them for creating a feeling that pregnancy is not about being hidden in a shelter and is a phase to be enjoyed. However, it should not be done at the cost of one's health, right? Can you name one influencer who had a very low lying placenta and she could travel to Europe? No, right? So, whatever we show on Instagram/Facebook should come with a disclaimer, 'please consider your medical conditions and seek doctor's advice before indulging in any adventurous activities'. This is because those who couldn't travel or even walk feel depressed about being isolated.

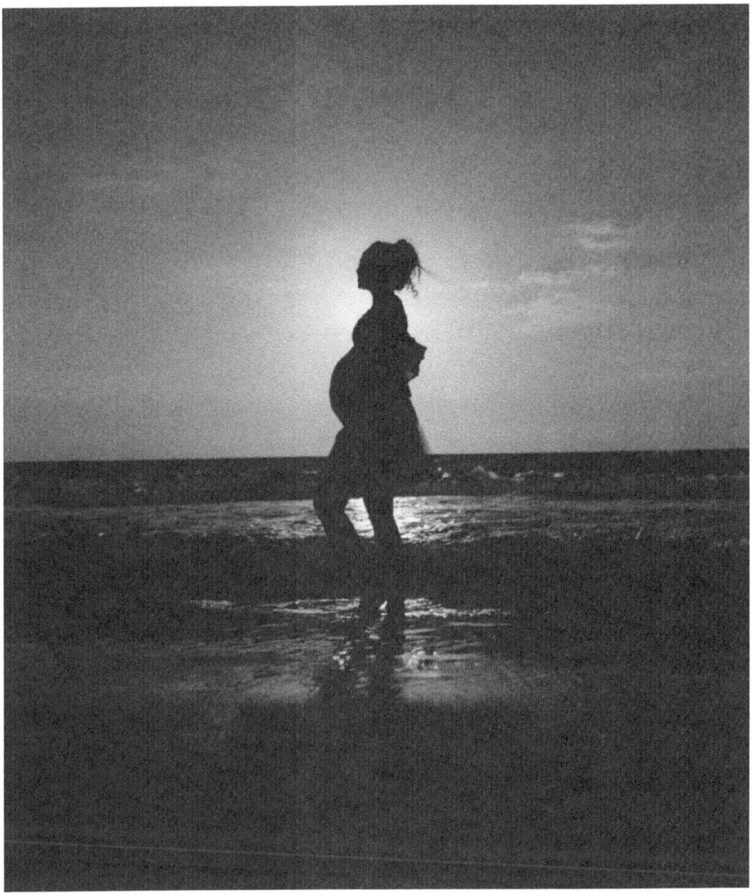

Among those watching from the side-lines is Parvartika, a hardworking and ambitious woman who once traveled the world for her job. However, her pregnancy journey has been far from smooth sailing. Complications have restricted her movements, forcing her to set aside her adventurous lifestyle and prioritize her health and that of her unborn child. Parvartika was a little overweight and she had a family history of diabetes. She had a small cervix and she had that stitched last week. She has been almost on bed rest for the last 5 days.

As Parvartika scrolls through her social media feed, she can't help but feel a pang of envy and disappointment. She sees influencers and celebrities jetting off to exotic destinations for their babymoons, showing off their seemingly carefree pregnancies, and effortlessly balancing their glamorous careers with impending motherhood.

While Parvartika appreciates and respects the women who can embrace their pregnancies in this way, she also recognizes the stark difference between their experiences and hers. As a middle-class woman without a support system or access to high-class treatments, she grapples with the reality that her journey is far from the picture-perfect image portrayed on social media.

The glitzy portrayals of pregnancy on social media can be both inspiring and demoralizing. While it's empowering to witness women embracing their pregnancies and celebrating motherhood, it can also inadvertently create feelings of inadequacy and guilt for those who cannot mirror the same experiences.

Parvartika often wonders if she is doing something wrong or if she should be pushing herself harder to be more like the influencers she sees online. The pressure to keep up with the glamorous standards set by social media can be overwhelming, leaving her feeling anxious and insecure about her own journey.

The truth is that every pregnancy is unique, and each woman's experience is shaped by various factors such as health, financial situation, support network, and individual circumstances. Comparing one's journey to the carefully curated highlight reels on social media can lead to unrealistic expectations and unnecessary self-criticism.

It's important to remember that social media offers only a glimpse into people's lives, often presenting an idealized version rather than the full reality. The influencers and celebrities may indeed be experiencing smooth pregnancies, but it doesn't invalidate the challenges faced by others like Parvartika.

Parvartika spoke to her friend Supriya, "How can someone dive into water, visit multiple places, and look so glowy all the while in pregnancy?"

Supriya was her friend and has been with her for the last 2 years, "And here I am looking like a cow, I have no energy left to even go to the office."

"Exactly, all of this portrayed on social media is not 100% true, because they have access to good food, financial support, and good house help. But this portrayal generates a fair amount of expectations in a middle-class family. These influencers can even travel to countries during their pregnancies, but you can't even go to the office?", replied Parvartika.

"Yes, they should definitely put out a disclaimer saying, 'I could do all these shoots, travel, heavy lifting because my body allowed me, and since every body is different, one should take care of their body and baby first", told Supriya.

"Absolutely, one day my office colleague was making fun of my walk, and then he pointed out to some influencers doing a ramp walk gracefully during pregnancy. He didn't even realize that the penguin walk became normal for me because earning just 30000 per month, I cannot afford a highly nutritious diet and super classy footwear to keep my walk toned.

Author says in a country like India, where women lack basic nutritious food in pregnancy ; **we must create awareness about that healthy eating and healthy exercises** first. According to Mint article dated, 18 Nov 2019, 08:29 PM IST *https://www.livemint.com/science/health/less-than-half-of-*

the-pregnant-women-in-rural-india-get-nutritious-food-survey-11574089051372.html.

New Delhi: Less than half of pregnant women in rural India eat nutritious food, and the majority are deprived of quality healthcare, as revealed by an independent survey conducted by three researchers associated with the Indian Institute of Management-Ahmedabad and Ranchi University.

The survey, titled Jaccha-Baccha Survey (JABS), was carried out by Jean Dreze, a professor at Ranchi University, Reetika Khera, an associate professor at IIM Ahmedabad, and Anmol Somanchi, a research associate with IIM-A, across six states: Chhattisgarh, Himachal Pradesh, Jharkhand, Madhya Pradesh, Odisha, and Uttar Pradesh.

In each state, the survey teams visited 10-12 randomly selected anganwadis (spread over two blocks in the same district) and interviewed as many pregnant and nursing women registered at those anganwadis as possible, totaling 342 and 364 respondents, respectively.

According to the survey, only 22% of nursing women reported eating more than usual during their pregnancy, and merely 31% claimed to have consumed more nutritious food than usual. The primary reason for not eating more is that many pregnant women feel unwell or experience a loss of appetite. The proportion of nursing women who reported eating nutritious food (such as eggs, fish, and milk) "regularly" during pregnancy was less than half in the entire sample, and just 12% in Uttar Pradesh.

"Poor diets lead to low weight gain during pregnancy. Compared with a norm of 13-18 kg for women with low BMI, the average weight gain in the sample was barely 7 kg (in UP, just 4 kg). Pregnant and nursing women are acutely deprived of quality healthcare. Many of them receive some basic services (such as tetanus injections and iron tablets) at

the local anganwadi or health center, but they get very little beyond the basics," said Khera.

"Minor ailments can easily become a major burden in terms of pain or expenses or both. At the time of delivery, women are often sent to private hospitals when there are complications. A significant minority also report rude, hostile, or even brutal treatment in the labor room," she added.

As Parvartika continues her pregnancy journey, she finds solace in the stories of other women who have faced similar challenges. She discovers online communities that share honest and unfiltered accounts of pregnancy, offering a more balanced and realistic perspective. She has joined several WhatsApp and Telegram groups.

Through these platforms, Parvartika connects with women from different backgrounds who have navigated their own unique paths through pregnancy. She learns that it's okay to prioritize her well-being and the well-being of her child, even if it means sacrificing certain experiences that others might enjoy.

Parvartika realizes that her worth as a mother and a woman is not determined by her ability to mimic the lives of influencers on social media. Her journey is authentic and courageous, filled with resilience and love for her unborn child.

In the end, Parvartika embraces the duality of pregnancy on social media. She acknowledges the allure and inspiration it can offer while understanding the importance of filtering through the glamour to find authenticity.

Her experience serves as a reminder that social media should be taken with a grain of salt, and it's essential to focus on one's journey rather than comparing it to others. Each woman's pregnancy is a unique and beautiful chapter, and it's vital to celebrate the individuality and strength that lies within every expectant mother.

As Parvartika continues to navigate her pregnancy journey, she realizes that embracing her own truth and being authentic is more empowering than trying to live up to societal expectations or social media standards.

She learns to set boundaries for herself, knowing when to disconnect from the pressures of the online world and focus on her well-being and that of her unborn child.

Throughout her pregnancy, Parvartika finds support from unexpected places. Strangers in online communities become her confidants, offering empathy and understanding. She discovers that she is not alone in feeling the weight of societal pressures and that there is strength in vulnerability and seeking support.

Parvartika's closest friends and family rally around her, acknowledging her struggles and championing her strength. They remind her that her pregnancy journey is not defined by the glamorous images on social media but by the love, resilience, and sacrifices she makes for her child.

In a world where comparison and self-doubt can run rampant, Parvartika chooses to be her advocate and champion. She embraces her journey, recognizing that her experiences are no less valid or beautiful than those glamorized on social media.

The birth of Parvartika's child brings a new wave of strength and purpose. As she holds her baby in her arms, she knows that she has weathered the storm of societal pressures and emerged stronger and more self-assured.

During a beautiful rainy season with black clouds hovering around, she sips a cup of coffee while watching reels from her balcony. Dressed in loose-fitting pajamas and a high messy bun, Parvartika realizes it's time to change the thought process.

She then takes to Instagram and starts sharing her authentic journey of pregnancy. She writes about how she truly feels and describes her complications. In a world where complications are not often discussed, she shares her stories about cervix stitches and low-lying placenta. She shares her story not to seek validation but to empower and support women who may feel overlooked or misunderstood in their own pregnancy journeys.

Through her candidness and vulnerability, Parvartika fosters a sense of community and acceptance among women. She encourages open conversations about the challenges and triumphs of motherhood, breaking the barrier of judgment and unrealistic expectations set by social media.

Over time, Parvartika's advocacy for authentic representation of pregnancy on social media gains momentum. She collaborates with other mothers and influencers to create a space that celebrates all pregnancy experiences, free from the confines of comparison and judgment.

Parvartika's movement sparks a change in the way society perceives and supports pregnant women. The emphasis shifts from glamorizing experiences to embracing the diverse and unique journeys each woman embarks on.

As the years passed, the influence of Parvartika's movement reached far and wide. Expectant mothers from all parts of India found comfort in knowing that their experiences were valid and worthy of celebration, regardless of how they aligned with social media trends. Parvartika's legacy extended beyond her online presence. In her local community, she created support groups for pregnant women, providing a safe space for them to share their stories and seek advice without judgment.

Here are some of the comments/conversations that made headlines in the community:

There were a few examples of how pregnant women might express negativity when comparing themselves to influencers who seem to stay fit, travel, and maintain a "glowy" appearance during pregnancy:

"I constantly see these influencers looking perfect and active throughout their pregnancies. Meanwhile, I struggle with morning sickness and fatigue. It's hard not to feel like I'm failing somehow."

"Seeing influencers effortlessly working out and flaunting their baby bumps makes me feel inadequate. I can barely keep up with daily activities and office work, let alone intense workouts at the gym. I can only do a 1-hour exercise at home."

"It's frustrating to see influencers traveling to exotic locations and attending events while pregnant. I'm stuck dealing with discomfort and unable to do most of the things I used to enjoy because of my complications."

"I feel guilty for not looking as 'glowy' as these influencers. My skin is breaking out, and I have stretch marks. It's like I'm not living up to the pregnancy beauty standards."

"I'm constantly bombarded by these images of women who seem to effortlessly manage their careers, fitness routines, and pregnancy. Meanwhile, I struggle to concentrate at work and sometimes just want to rest."

"It's hard not to compare myself to these influencers who are always camera-ready. My hair is a mess, I feel bloated, and I'm not sure how to feel good about myself right now."

"Seeing influencers talk about their active pregnancies and watching them do yoga poses with a baby bump makes me feel like I'm not doing enough. I wish I had their energy and flexibility."

"I'm dealing with constant nausea and exhaustion, and seeing influencers talk about how wonderful pregnancy is can be disheartening. I wish I felt as glowing and positive as they seem."

"I know social media isn't reality, but it's hard not to feel bad when influencers post about their 'perfect' pregnancies. Meanwhile, I'm dealing with mood swings and hormonal changes that make me feel like a mess."

"Comparing myself to influencers who document their picture-perfect pregnancies only adds to my stress. I don't feel like I'm measuring up to their standards, and it's affecting my self-esteem."

These quotes highlighted the range of emotions and thoughts that pregnant women might experience when they perceive a gap between their own pregnancy experiences and the curated portrayal of influencers on social media. It's important for pregnant women to prioritize their well-being and focus on their own unique journey, seeking support when needed and practicing self-compassion.

Through her advocacy and compassionate nature, Parvartika transformed the perception of pregnancy in her society. She became a source of inspiration for women to embrace their journeys with confidence and self-assurance.

In the end, Parvartika's story is a testament to the power of authenticity and empathy. It teaches us that the beauty of pregnancy lies not in how it is perceived on social media but in the strength, love, and resilience displayed by every expectant mother, regardless of their circumstances.

As Parvartika continued her journey of advocating for authentic representation of pregnancy on social media, she came across a common misconception prevalent in society - the idea that traveling and enjoying pregnancy is solely a result of hard work and dedication.

Through her own experiences and conversations with other expectant mothers, Parvartika realized that the ability to travel and enjoy pregnancy to the fullest is sometimes a matter of luck and privilege. Pregnancy complications can arise unexpectedly, affecting a woman's mobility and energy levels. This may prevent her from engaging in certain activities or traveling, regardless of her dedication and ambition. Furthermore, the financial aspect plays a significant role in a pregnant woman's ability to access additional help and support. Those with sufficient financial resources can afford to hire household help, childcare, or even personal medical assistance, making their pregnancy experience more manageable.

On the other hand, middle-class women like Parvartika often find themselves balancing multiple responsibilities without access to additional support. The lack of financial resources and help can be a significant barrier to fully enjoying the pregnancy journey. As she delved deeper into this issue, Parvartika realized that the glamorized portrayal of pregnancy on social media often perpetuates unrealistic standards. Many influencers and celebrities have the privilege of financial stability and assistance, which enables them to travel, work, and enjoy their pregnancies without the same challenges faced by others.

It became evident to Parvartika that pregnancy experiences are not homogenous. They are shaped by an individual's health, financial status, support network, and sheer luck of not encountering severe complications.

Parvartika sought to dismantle the notion that hard work and dedication are the sole factors influencing a smooth pregnancy journey. Instead, she emphasized the importance of acknowledging the role luck and privilege play in shaping each woman's experience.

Through her advocacy, Parvartika encouraged women to embrace their journeys authentically, without feeling pressured to conform to societal expectations based on social media portrayals. She emphasized that every pregnancy, irrespective of the ability to travel or enjoy certain activities, is a unique and valuable experience that deserves celebration and support.

Parvartika's message resonated with many expectant mothers who had previously felt inadequate due to the unrealistic standards perpetuated by social media. As her movement gained momentum, more women began sharing their own unfiltered and honest pregnancy experiences, highlighting the diversity and individuality of each journey.

What should influencers do?

Yes, we agree that it takes a lot of courage to do exercises, go to shoots while gracefully managing pregnancy, and travel during pregnancy, and the author really thanks the influencers for building an inspiring society.

However, the posts should come with a disclaimer that it is advisable to consult your doctor and consider your health conditions first before involving yourself in any activities mentioned above.

CHAPTER 6

CHALLENGING MISINTERPRETATIONS

In the bustling household of the Raghavi family, Mrs. Raghavi finds herself navigating the challenges of pregnancy, both physical and emotional. Her doctor advises her to stay active during this time, emphasizing the importance of maintaining a healthy lifestyle.

On a bustling busy morning, Raghavi went to Motherkid Hospital with her husband. There was a huge rush as it was the weekend. Next to the waiting room, there was a labor room, and Raghavi saw a patient being wheeled in on a stretcher. A reception desk was at the center, with the stem cell storage counter next to it, and a prominently white wall adorned with images of children. She was waiting for her doctor to arrive, feeling anxious about the instructions from the doctor. She was wearing a red maternity gown and looked beautiful with her long hair parted on both sides. Her sandals were causing discomfort as her feet were badly swollen.

The doctor had asked them to wait as she was in the Operation Theatre (OT). Raghavi walked around to ease her anxiety. Then, the doctor arrived with an OT gown and headwear, in a hurry due to the long queue of patients outside her cabin.

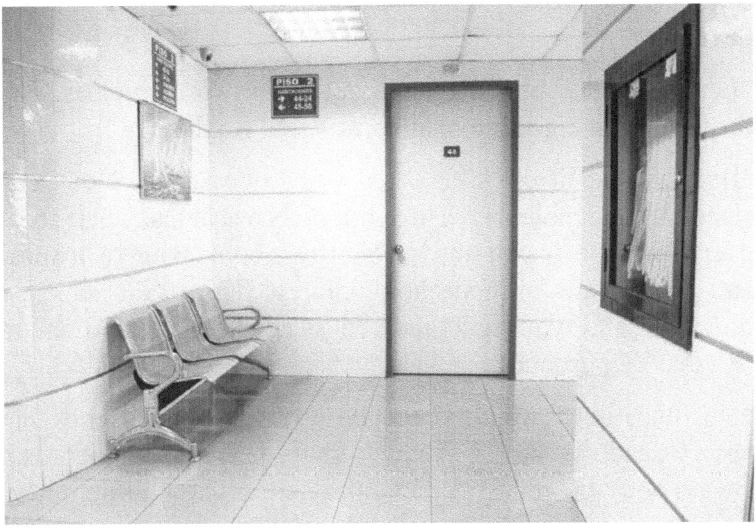

After three patients, Raghavi's turn came.

"How are you doing, Raghavi?" Dr. Leena asked.

"Yes, ma'am, I am doing great, but I have pain in my back and heartburn is not letting me eat anything. Also, with the swollen feet, I feel I can't even walk, so I try to avoid walking," replied Raghavi.

"Beta, you will have to stay active, keep walking, engage yourself in some activities that freshen up your mind," Dr. Leena said.

"Sure, Ma'am, I will start doing exercises and will start walking," said Mrs. Raghavi.

"I am prescribing Folic acid and Calcium. Continue taking them on time. Your ultrasound report looks perfectly fine. The baby is healthy," Dr. Leena insisted.

"Next patient please," Dr. Leena asked her secretary.

Mrs. Raghavi and her husband thanked the doctor and left the cabin.

"Let's go to the pharmacy and get these two medicines. The doctor has changed the medicines," said Raghavi.

"But did you listen? She asked you to be active. You keep sleeping the whole day. There are other ways also apart from exercise to keep you active. You can cook your own meal and participate in household chores. This will help my mumma, and you will also be benefitted," told Jitendra (Raghavi's husband).

"No Jitu, I don't want to engage myself in any activities that have a deadline. It creates unnecessary pressure on me. Also, I want activities that fill me with positivity. I will definitely do some household chores and help your mumma, but I won't commit to doing it every day like I do for my exercise. I can't even do exercises every day. I do them at my own convenience and at a comfortable time," replied Raghavi.

"You ladies just drag things. I really don't understand your so-called 'logics,' ever," Jitendra vented out.

However, as often happens in many households, the statement "stay active" is misinterpreted by husbands and mothers-in-law. They firmly believe that the only way for a woman to stay active is by engaging in household chores, particularly in the kitchen.

Raghavi, who is already feeling the weight of pregnancy and the emotional rollercoaster that comes with it, is now burdened with additional responsibilities in the kitchen.

Despite expressing her discomfort, her husband and mother-in-law insist that she must follow the doctor's advice.

In reality, the doctor's advice to "stay active" was intended to encourage Raghavi to engage in light physical activities, such as walking, stretching, or prenatal exercises, that suit her individual comfort and energy levels.

Misinterpretations of medical advice are not uncommon, and in Raghavi's case, it leads to increased stress and frustration during her pregnancy journey.

She longs for her husband and mother-in-law to understand her perspective, to acknowledge that her pregnancy journey is unique, and that what she needs most right now is love, support, and understanding.

Amidst her struggle, Raghavi pays a visit to her doctor, hoping to gain some clarity and guidance. The doctor reassures her that her feelings are valid and that every pregnancy comes with its own set of challenges.

The doctor emphasizes the importance of self-care and self-compassion during pregnancy. She encourages Raghavi to prioritize her well-being and happiness, even if it means taking a step back from certain household responsibilities.

As the days go by, Raghavi's frustration grows, and she starts to feel increasingly isolated in her own home. Her husband and mother-in-law continue to push her to work in the kitchen, believing that it is the only way for her to stay active during pregnancy.

The pressure and stress from the misinterpretation of the doctor's advice take a toll on Raghavi's mental and emotional well-being. She finds herself constantly second-guessing her own feelings and questioning whether she is being unreasonable.

Here are some examples of how doctor's advice about staying active and healthy during pregnancy might be misinterpreted by family members and in-laws, leading to potential trouble for pregnant women:

Excessive Chores: Misinterpretation: "Staying active means keeping up with household chores like before." Family members might expect the pregnant woman to continue with her usual chores, leading to exhaustion and potential health issues.

Social Expectations: Misinterpretation: "Staying healthy means attending all family events and gatherings." Family members might pressure the pregnant woman to participate in social events even if she needs rest or is uncomfortable.

Traditional Restrictions: Misinterpretation: "Staying healthy means following traditional dietary restrictions strictly." Overemphasis on traditional practices might lead to a lack of essential nutrients needed for the pregnant woman's health.

Lack of Rest: Misinterpretation: "Staying active means no need for extra rest." Family members might discourage rest or suggest it's unnecessary, leading to fatigue and stress for the pregnant woman.

Work and Financial Pressure: Misinterpretation: "Staying active means continuing to work as usual." Family members might prioritize financial concerns over the woman's health, causing physical and emotional strain.

Intrusive Advice: Misinterpretation: "Staying healthy means following every piece of advice from family members." Unsolicited advice from family members might lead to conflicting information and increased stress.

Ignoring Doctor's Recommendations: Misinterpretation: "Family wisdom is more valuable than doctor's advice." In-laws or older family members might dismiss modern medical advice, leading to potential health risks.

Comparison to Others: Misinterpretation: "Other pregnant women manage fine, so should you." Unreasonable comparisons can lead to emotional distress and the woman feeling pressured to meet unrealistic standards.

Inadequate Support: Misinterpretation: "You're fine on your own, you don't need extra support." Lack of emotional and physical support from family members can lead to isolation and stress.

Misguided Nutrition: Misinterpretation: "Staying healthy means eating whatever family members suggest." Following family dietary recommendations without considering medical advice can lead to nutritional imbalances.

Disregarding Rest Signs: Misinterpretation: "Resting is laziness." Family members might equate resting with laziness, leading the pregnant woman to ignore her body's signals and overexert herself.

Emotional Pressure: Misinterpretation: "Staying healthy means not expressing negative emotions." Family members might discourage expressing emotions, potentially impacting the woman's mental health.

Her husband and mother-in-law, initially taken aback, dismiss her concerns and tell her that she is overthinking and exaggerating the situation. They believe that they know what's best for her and that she should follow their advice without questioning.

This dismissal of her feelings makes Raghavi feel unheard and unimportant. She struggles to express her needs, fearing that she will be labeled as dramatic or difficult.

As Raghavi's due date approaches, she reflects on the journey she has been through—the joy, the struggles, and the misinterpretations. She realizes that she has been silenced and disregarded for far too long.

In moments of vulnerability, Raghavi confides in her close friends and finds solace in their understanding and support. They validate her feelings and remind her that her needs and comfort should be the top priority during pregnancy.

As Raghavi's pregnancy progressed, she couldn't help but notice how her friends and other expectant mothers were being cared for and supported by their families. Her best friend, Priya, who was also pregnant, had a completely different experience. Priya's husband and in-laws were attentive to her needs, ensuring she rested when required and offering to help with household chores.

Seeing this contrast, Raghavi couldn't help but feel a pang of sadness and longing. She yearned for the same level of care and support from her own family, but her husband and mother-in-law remained adamant in their belief that she should continue working in the kitchen despite her pregnancy.

On one occasion, when Raghavi tried to attend a prenatal yoga session, her mother-in-law looked down upon her decision. She told Raghavi's husband that "there was no need for her to attend such classes because all the benefits could be obtained by working in the house, cleaning, and washing. These small exercises are already part of Kitchen chores."

Raghavi felt hurt and unsupported, as she knew that prenatal yoga offered much more than just physical benefits. It was an opportunity for her to connect with her body, her baby, and find moments of relaxation and mindfulness during the emotional rollercoaster of pregnancy.

"Ma, kitchen work doesn't give me positivity, but exercises do. Why can't you understand this mere difference? I feel exhausted when I work in the kitchen. I slog from 7 am in the morning till 10 am to prepare food for both of you. And apart from this, you expect me to clean and sweep floors. How on earth is that logical?" asked Raghavi.

"Duck walk these days is the same as sweeping the floor. The Malasana these days is the same as using Indian toilets. The Chakki Chalan in your prenatal exercise is the actual Chakki chalan from our days. The cat and cow pose is almost the same as brooming the floor. And we never thought of these chores as negative. We couldn't even reply back to my Mother in law," replied her MIL.

"Okay, did you go to the office also? Did you attend meetings as well while you had to pee? Did you sleep in the afternoon? And how about food? You had access to clean and unaltered food. The environment was not polluted like here in Delhi. You had a child when you were 19, I am delivering at 29. Can't you see the differences in generations? Can you not see me taking care of the office with utmost efficiency?" replied Raghavi in a stern tone.

Despite her body sending signals to slow down and rest, Raghavi was forced to continue working until her seventh month of pregnancy. The physical strain and emotional stress became overwhelming, and one fateful day, Raghavi experienced premature contractions. Terrified and in pain, Raghavi was rushed to the hospital, where the doctors worked tirelessly to prevent an early delivery. It was a wake-up call for her husband and mother-in-law, who finally realized the severity of their actions and the impact it had on Raghavi's health.

In the hospital room, as Raghavi lay on the bed, she couldn't help but feel a mix of anger and sadness. She wished she had been heard, that her needs had been respected, and that her family had understood the significance of taking care of a pregnant woman.

It was a turning point for Raghavi's husband and mother-in-law. Seeing her in distress, they vowed to change their approach and prioritize her well-being. They understood that being active during pregnancy did not mean overexerting oneself in household chores but rather finding a balance that suited her comfort and energy levels.

As Raghavi recovered in the hospital, her husband took on more responsibilities at home and sought the help of a housekeeper. He realized that hiring help was a small price to pay for ensuring Raghavi's health and the well-being of their unborn child.

With the doctor's words resonating in her heart, Raghavi decides to have an open and honest conversation with her husband and mother-in-law. She explains the toll that the misinterpretation of the doctor's advice took on her and expresses her need for empathy and understanding.

With newfound determination, Raghavi mustered the courage to speak up once more. In a heartfelt and assertive manner, she shares her feelings of being misunderstood and undervalued during her pregnancy journey. She explains that her needs and well-being should be respected, and she should have the freedom to decide which activities make her feel comfortable and active. To her surprise, her husband and mother-in-law initially resist her words, but this time, Raghavi stands her ground. She refuses to be silenced any longer and demands the respect and empathy she deserves.

In conclusion, Raghavi's story is a testament to the power of speaking up and advocating for one's needs. It showcases the significance of understanding and empathy during pregnancy and the importance of breaking free from societal expectations.

Let us remember that every woman's pregnancy journey is unique and deserves to be honored and respected. As a society, let us champion the importance of creating a supportive and inclusive environment for all expectant mothers, where they feel heard, valued, and cherished throughout this beautiful and transformative journey of motherhood.

CHAPTER 7
DOUBLE THE TROUBLE

Once upon a time, in a bustling city, there lived a young woman named Alka. She was a determined and ambitious individual who had always strived for success in both her personal and professional life. Alka was happily married, and to her delight, she discovered that she was expecting a child. However, as the days passed, Alka realized that navigating the journey of a working pregnant woman in the modern world was far more challenging than she had ever imagined. She had to go to the office every day and manage household chores as well.

The days started blending together as Alka worked relentlessly from home. She had envisioned this time to be filled with joy and excitement, but it felt like a never-ending struggle. Nausea, leg pain, and backspin haunted her every moment, making it difficult to find solace even in her own home. The continuous virtual meetings and the relentless pressure to meet deadlines only added to her distress. She felt like her body was betraying her, preventing her from giving her best at work.

As weeks turned into months, Alka's exhaustion grew, and she found herself caught in an unrelenting cycle. There was no escape, no break, and no moment to catch her breath. She yearned for some respite, but the demands of work seemed to engulf every aspect of her life. The inability to take proper breaks or enjoy freshly prepared meals added to her frustration and sense of helplessness.

When Alka received news that she had to return to the office a few days a week, it felt like a crushing blow. The thought of commuting 15 kms every day while being pregnant seemed daunting, and she feared her body would succumb to the stress of it all. Still, she had no choice but to comply with her employer's demands. After all, she had to take Maternity leave, and changing jobs at this point would not make any sense. The days she spent in the office were even more challenging. She struggled to focus on her work, distracted by the constant discomfort and the overwhelming urge to rest.

Alka's colleagues seemed oblivious to her struggles, and she felt isolated, battling her demons silently. She tried to remain calm and composed in the office, afraid of being judged or perceived as weak. The weight of it all became unbearable, but she wore a facade of strength, hiding her pain and fears behind a brave smile.

As the days turned into months, Alka's once vibrant spirit began to wither under the weight of her relentless responsibilities. The constant demands of her job and the ever-present struggles of her pregnancy seemed to be closing in on her, suffocating her dreams and aspirations. What was meant to be a joyous time of anticipation and excitement had turned into an arduous journey of endurance, leaving her feeling utterly defeated.

One of the most challenging aspects was the struggle to maintain a balanced and nutritious diet. Due to the demands of her job and the lack of flexibility, Alka often found herself skipping meals or relying on quick and unhealthy snacks to keep her going. The lack of freshly prepared food not only affected her physical health but also took a toll on her mental well-being, leaving her feeling guilty and anxious about the impact on her unborn child.

Each day, as the clock ticked away, Alka's lunchtime became a distant memory, buried under piles of work and pressing deadlines. She would stare at the clock, longing for a moment to nourish her body, but her responsibilities seemed to override her basic needs. She didn't get time to touch her belly and talk to her baby. This constant neglect of her health weighed heavily on her conscience, as she feared the consequences it might have on the growth and development of her baby.

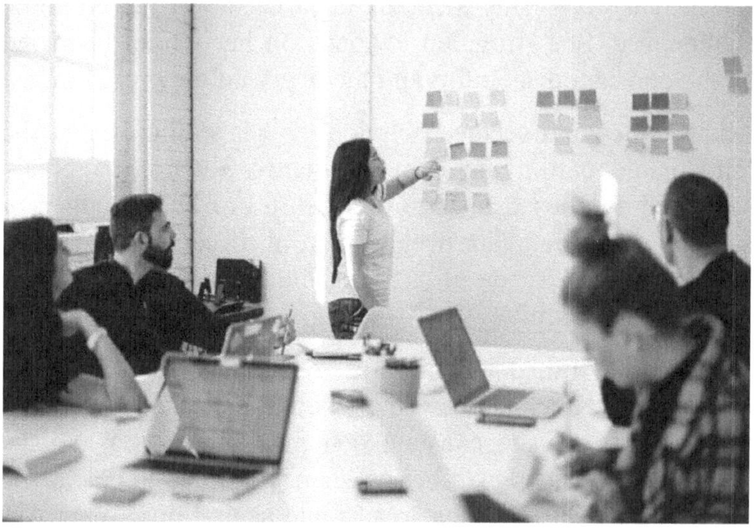

Another challenge that Alka faced was the struggle to take her medications on time. Amidst the chaos of her work and household responsibilities, she often forgot to take the prenatal vitamins prescribed by her doctor. Each missed dose added to her stress, as she worried about the potential impact on her baby's health. However, admitting her oversight to her doctor felt like acknowledging her failure as a responsible mother-to-be.

The days Alka spent in the office were no less trying. The daily commute exposed her to the bustling city streets, filled with dust and pollution. The crowded public transport and the constant rush of people left her feeling vulnerable and overwhelmed. Each breath she took felt heavy with pollutants, and she worried about the potential harm it might cause to her unborn child. She used to monitor baby movements not in hope but in apprehension.

The office environment, too, presented its own set of challenges. The air-conditioned rooms, though a respite from the scorching sun outside, left Alka feeling cold and uncomfortable. Her migraine also came back that was subsided a few years ago. Yet, she hesitated to speak up about her discomfort, not wanting to draw attention to her pregnancy and appear weak or incapable in the eyes of her colleagues.

During her commute and the time spent outdoors, Alka could feel the impact on her health, with bouts of sneezing and nasal congestion becoming a regular occurrence. The fear of falling sick loomed over her, as she knew that getting ill could pose further risks to her pregnancy.

Despite the challenges, Alka pressed on, determined to fulfill her responsibilities both at work and home. The frustration and exhaustion she felt were often masked behind a facade of strength and composure, as she didn't want her loved ones to worry about her. Yet, as the days passed, the toll on her mental and physical health became evident, leaving her feeling drained and defeated.

On certain days, when Alka finally returned home, covered in dust and fatigue, she could barely summon the energy to do the simplest of household chores. The exhaustion was overwhelming, and she longed for a moment of peace and rest. Yet, the responsibilities of managing the household and preparing meals beckoned, leaving her with little time to relax and rejuvenate.

As her health deteriorated, Alka's body seemed to be rebelling against her. The nausea that once visited her in the mornings now lingered throughout the day, making it a constant battle to keep even the smallest meals down. The frequent leg pain and backspin made it difficult for her to stand, and she often found herself clutching onto nearby surfaces for support to stand or even walk. The physical toll of pregnancy was exacerbated by the relentless demands of her job, leaving her feeling depleted and exhausted.

Despite her best efforts to remain strong, Alka's frustration grew with each passing day. She felt like she was being pulled in a million different directions, trying to fulfill the expectations of her employer, her family, and herself. The sense of being trapped in a never-ending cycle was suffocating, and she yearned for a moment of respite, a brief pause to catch her breath.

Every night, as she lay in bed, Alka felt a wave of sadness wash over her. She was haunted by the fear that she was failing as a mother before her child even arrived. She could not join prenatal exercises anymore, she could not invest time in worship, and even eating a full meal was a challenge. The guilt gnawed at her, consuming her thoughts, as she questioned her ability to provide the best environment for her baby amidst the chaos and exhaustion.

Despite her immense struggles, Alka remained silent about her frustrations, unwilling to burden her loved ones with her pain. She put on a brave face, concealing her inner turmoil behind a facade of strength. It became a lonely battle, and she found herself withdrawing from those around her, afraid that her vulnerability would be perceived as weakness.

As the months passed, Alka's health deteriorated further, and her doctor expressed concerns about the toll her high-stress lifestyle was taking on her and her unborn child. But leaving her job was not an option; she needed the income and felt a sense of responsibility to prove herself in the competitive work environment. She felt trapped, torn between her duties as a mother and her ambition to succeed in her career.

Alka's breaking point finally arrived. One evening, after a particularly challenging day at the office, Alka broke down in tears. She confided in her husband about her struggles and fears, and he could see the toll it was taking on her. He reassured her that she was not alone and encouraged her to prioritize her health and their baby's well-being above everything else.

The exhaustion had reached its peak, and she found herself unable to get out of bed. Her husband, worried and desperate to help, sat by her side, urging her to share her burdens. Through tear-filled eyes, she poured out her heart, revealing the depth of her frustration and fears. Her husband listened with empathy, his heart breaking for the woman he loved.

He told her husband, "My frustration is growing each day, and I feel trapped in a never-ending cycle of work and responsibilities. My health has started deteriorating, and I find it increasingly difficult to cope with the demands of my job and my pregnancy. It feels like I am failing as a mother before my child even arrives".

"Don't continue this. You have 26 earned leaves left. Take those leaves first and rest up for 1.5 months, and as per the legal clause, nobody can fire you on the pretext of pregnancy. During leave, support your office while working from home," replied Sanjay (Alka's husband).

"Yes, let me talk to Ashok (my manager) and get this approved, but will this not affect my goodwill? And everyone will call me an excuse maker," replied Alka.

"Let them call, what is more important today, your health or other's validations? You need to choose one path for yourself. Also, you are not denying any work. You are still one of the best employees, and Ashok will understand your feelings," told Sanjay.

With unwavering support and love, Alka's husband encouraged her to prioritize her health and their child's well-being above all else. He reassured her that her worth was not defined by her job or her ability to be the perfect working woman. He reminded her that being a mother was already a feat of strength and resilience, and she had nothing to prove to anyone.

In that moment, Alka realized that she had been neglecting her own needs, sacrificing her well-being for the sake of others' expectations. She understood that her happiness and the well-being of her baby should take precedence over any professional achievements. With newfound clarity, she made a difficult decision to step back from her demanding job and focus on taking care of herself and her unborn child.

CHAPTER 8

C-SECTION VS NORMAL DELIVERY

The journey begins in a quaint little town, where Lavanya and Parineeta were both expecting their first child. Lavanya, a career-oriented woman with curly hair and a youthful appearance, was in her early thirties. She had meticulously planned her pregnancy and eagerly awaited the arrival of her baby. She did all her prenatal exercises on time and maintained a very healthy eating habit since the first month of her pregnancy. Parineeta, on the other hand, was lean and could only exercise until her eighth month. She had a fondness for eating junk food, had a more laid-back attitude, and took things as they came. Both women were overjoyed at the prospect of becoming mothers.

In the hospital rooms, Lavanya and Parineeta anxiously awaited the arrival of their children as the sun rose on a crisp morning, casting a pleasant warmth over them.

With her carefully thought-out birth plan, Lavanya had envisioned a straightforward and natural delivery. She had pictured herself ushering her child into the world with poise and tenacity. She used to say a prayer every day, "God, please let me go through a normal delivery, and I will do whatever it takes to support the vaginal delivery." Parineeta,

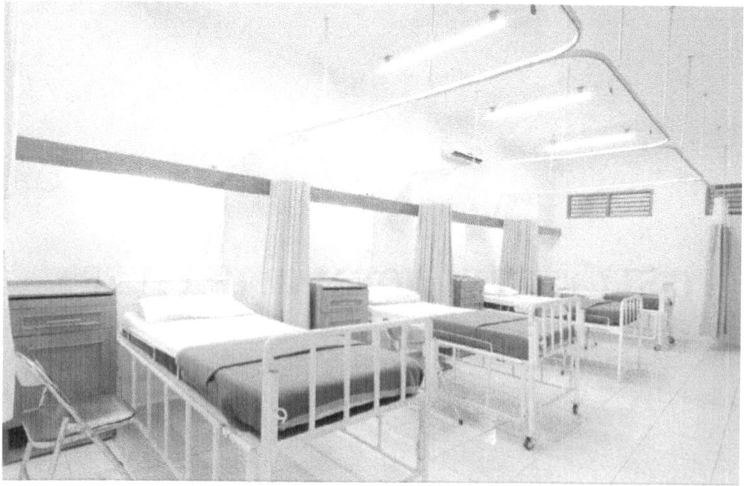

on the other hand, went into the day with a casual attitude and confidence in both her body and the laboring process. She never used to dwell on the delivery process, believing that whatever would happen was as per God's wish. The labor and delivery rooms buzzed with a mix of excitement and anxiety as contractions started for both women, about an hour apart. With the help of her husband and a group of supportive nurses, Parineeta concentrated on her breathing and surrendered to the rhythm of the contractions. She clutched her husband's wrist and cried out in pain.

In the room next door, Lavanya's journey took an unexpected turn. Her labor progressed rapidly, but her baby was not responding well to the stress of childbirth. The medical team, in consultation with her doctor, decided that an emergency c-section was the safest option for both Lavanya and the baby. Lavanya was taken aback by the sudden change in plans, her carefully crafted birth plan slipping through her fingers. Fear and uncertainty gripped Lavanya's heart as she was wheeled into the operating room. She had been expecting a normal delivery, and ending up in the operating room was one of her worst nightmares. The bright lights and sterile environment made her feel vulnerable and far from the serene atmosphere she had imagined. But amidst the whirlwind of emotions, the thought of soon holding her baby brought a glimmer of hope and excitement.

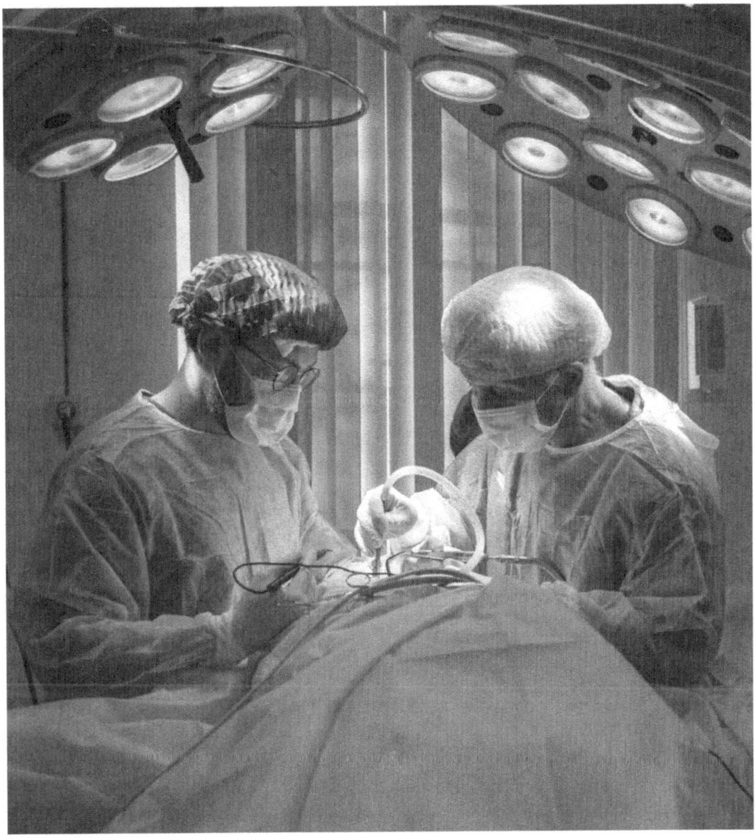

In the labor room next door, Parineeta's contractions intensified, and she felt a primal urge to push. Supported by her husband and the encouraging cheers of the nurses, she channeled her inner strength and pushed with all her might. Moments later, a cry filled the room, announcing the arrival of her precious bundle of joy. Tears of joy streamed down Parineeta's cheeks as she held her baby in her arms for the first time.

Meanwhile, in the operating room, Lavanya's heart raced as she awaited the moment she would meet her baby. The medical team worked swiftly, and soon she heard the sound of her baby's cries, a beautiful melody that brought tears of relief to her eyes. Both Lavanya and Parineeta had welcomed their little miracles into the world, but through different paths. Parineeta's delivery had been filled with the raw intensity of childbirth via natural delivery, while Lavanya's had been a rollercoaster of emotions, from carefully planned expectations to sudden twists and turns via c-section delivery.

As they were wheeled back to their hospital rooms, Lavanya and Parineeta felt a profound sense of accomplishment. Each had gone through a unique journey, discovering the depths of their strength and resilience in the process. Despite the challenges they faced, the love they felt for their babies was overwhelming, uniting them in a bond shared by all mothers.

As the initial euphoria of bringing their babies into the world settled, Lavanya and Parineeta found themselves facing the realities of postpartum recovery. Lavanya's c-section incision made even the simplest movements excruciatingly painful. Although she hadn't experienced labor pain because of the c-section, she was in extreme pain at this point. The pain medication provided some relief, but it came with its own set of side effects, leaving her feeling groggy and disconnected from the world. The lack of mobility was frustrating for Lavanya. As a fiercely independent woman, she had always prided herself on her ability to take care of herself. Now, she had to rely on her husband, Rishi, and the hospital staff to help with even the most basic tasks, like picking up her baby or getting out of bed.

Parineeta, too, found herself grappling with the physical toll of childbirth. The sleepless nights, combined with the demands of caring for a newborn, left her feeling utterly exhausted. Her body ached from the effort of breastfeeding and carrying her baby, and she often found herself nodding off during the day, only to be awakened by the cries of her hungry little one. But she had bypassed the labor pain, and she was recovering better than Lavanya because of the natural delivery.

Despite the challenges, Lavanya and Parineeta were determined to be the best mothers they could be. Their love for their babies overshadowed the weariness and pain they felt. Lavanya would gaze at her baby's tiny face and feel an overwhelming surge of love, making every ache and discomfort worth it. Parineeta would hold her baby close to her heart, finding solace in the warmth and connection they shared.

In the midst of their physical struggles, Lavanya and Parineeta found comfort in each other's company. They often sat together in the hospital room, sharing their stories of motherhood, laughter, and tears. Parineeta would offer Lavanya words of encouragement, reminding her that she was doing a fantastic job despite the challenges.

Lavanya, in turn, would marvel at Parineeta's carefree and positive attitude, finding inspiration in her friend's ability to embrace the unpredictability of motherhood. They leaned on each other for emotional support, knowing that they were the only ones who truly understood the rollercoaster of emotions they were experiencing.

As the days went by, Lavanya and Parineeta found themselves at the center of society's contrasting expectations for new mothers. Parineeta received an abundance of advice and compliments, with people admiring her for delivering her baby "naturally." Her mother-in-law said, "She showed a lot of courage, and only because of that, she could have a vaginal delivery." They lauded her for her bravery and endurance during the labor process. While Parineeta appreciated the support and kindness she received, she couldn't help but notice how society's focus on her method of delivery overshadowed other aspects of motherhood. The attention on her "normal" delivery seemed to elevate her in the eyes of some, almost as if her worth as a mother was directly linked to how her baby had come into the world.

On the other hand, Lavanya faced a different kind of scrutiny. She could feel the weight of judgmental glances and whispers that seemed to follow her whenever she mentioned her c-section delivery. People seemed quick to jump to conclusions, assuming that she had opted for the "easy way out." One day, at a gathering of new mothers, Lavanya overheard a group of women talking in hushed tones. "I can't believe she went for a c-section," one woman said, her tone filled with disdain. "I mean, didn't she even try for a normal delivery? It's like she didn't want to go through the real pain of childbirth. I also heard she used to do exercises. What are the benefits of investing in exercises when they can't guarantee a normal delivery?" Oblivious to the fact that a C-section or natural delivery process is based on the situation and not on someone's efforts. People who stay active and do exercises have a good chance of delivering naturally, but nobody can guarantee it. Not even doctors!

Hurt by the insensitive remarks, Lavanya felt a pang of self-doubt. She knew that her decision for a c-section was based on medical necessity, but she couldn't help but feel judged and misunderstood. It seemed as though society had boxed her into a narrow definition of what it meant to be a "strong" mother.

One evening, as Lavanya and Parineeta decided to meet, they chose a nice location in Hauz Khas. Both were looking a bit relaxed after enduring pain for the past few months and finally getting some time for themselves. They sat together and ordered a South Indian platter because they couldn't tolerate very spicy foods due to lactation. Lavanya opened up about her struggles with societal expectations. "It's just so unfair," Lavanya said, her voice trembling with emotion. "I feel like I have to constantly defend myself and explain why I had a c-section. As if my love for my baby is any less just because I didn't go through a natural delivery. The c-section took a toll on my health for 1.5 months, and I could not leave the house. How can someone call me weaker just because I had a c-section? Yes, I didn't feel the labor pain, but what I felt after delivery was no less than the delivery pain. The stitches pain, the back pain, the lack of mobility, and what not?"

Parineeta placed a comforting hand on Lavanya's shoulder.

"You don't owe anyone an explanation," she said firmly.

"Your journey as a mother is valid and beautiful, no matter how your baby came into this world. You made the best decision for you and your baby's health, and that's what matters the most."

Lavanya nodded, grateful for her friend's support.

"I just wish people would understand that every mother's journey is different," she said.

"We shouldn't be pitted against each other based on how we delivered our babies. We're all doing the best we can for our children."

Lavanya agreed wholeheartedly.

"You're absolutely right," she said.

"Motherhood is a journey of love, sacrifice, and resilience. It's not defined by how our babies are born but by the unconditional love we have for them."

The author asserts that we, as a society, should not be judgmental towards C-section moms and should not label them as weaker or tender. They may not endure the pain before or during delivery, but they do experience pain after delivery. For moms going through a normal delivery, they feel pain like bones cracking. Both these pains can't be compared, and they both come with different sets of pros and cons. We should respect women for bringing life into this world instead of scrutinizing their actions. Ultimately, every mother wants the best for her child.

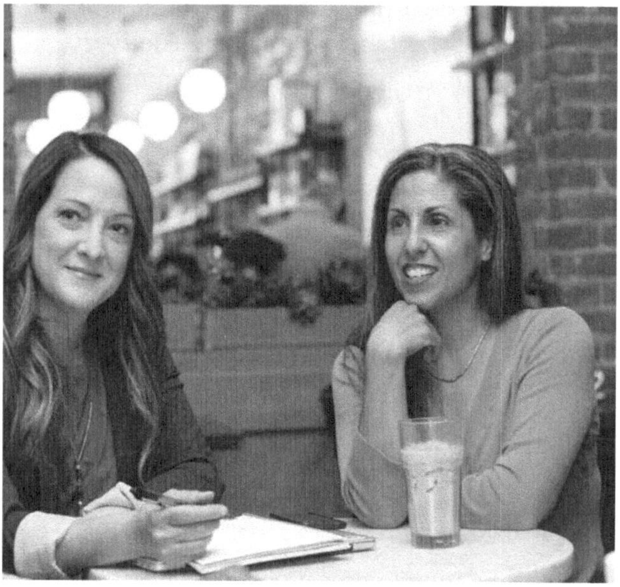

Now, let's talk about some examples of how women have expressed feelings of discrimination related to pregnancy, childbirth, and motherhood:

1. Online Testimonial: "I shared my C-section experience online, and I received comments about how I 'took the easy way out.' It hurt that people didn't understand the medical necessity behind my choice."

2. Conversation with Friends: "When my friends discussed childbirth experiences, they seemed to glorify natural birth and downplayed C-sections. I felt like my experience wasn't valued."

3. Workplace Conversation: "A co-worker told me I was lucky to get maternity leave and that I had 'vacation time' to relax. They didn't understand the physical and emotional toll of giving birth."

4. Family Gathering: "During a family gathering, my mother-in-law mentioned how quickly her generation bounced back after childbirth. I felt judged for not meeting those expectations as I took time to heal after C-section."

5. In-Laws' Comments: "My in-laws kept telling me to avoid C-section because 'real women' give birth naturally. It made me feel like I was less of a woman for needing medical assistance."

6. Pregnancy Fitness Class: "I joined a pregnancy fitness class, and the instructor focused only on vaginal births. I felt excluded and unsupported as a C-section mom-to-be."

7. Social Media Criticism: "After I shared my breastfeeding challenges online, I received comments about how C-section moms can't breastfeed properly. It was demoralizing."

8. Baby Care Workshop: "During a baby care workshop, the instructor praised vaginal birth for creating a stronger bond with the baby. I had a C-section, and it made me doubt my connection."

9. Job Promotion Discussion: "When I was up for a promotion, my boss questioned my commitment because I had taken maternity leave. It felt like discrimination based on my decision to have a family."

10. Community Gathering: "At a community event, other mothers discussed their childbirth stories. I felt isolated because I didn't have a 'natural' birth story to share."

11. Mother's Group Interaction: "In my mother's group, I was met with judgment when I mentioned formula feeding due to medical reasons. I felt like my choices were being scrutinized."

12. Hospital Experience: "During my stay at the hospital after a C-section, some nurses seemed less attentive because they assumed my experience was less 'serious' than a vaginal birth."

These examples highlight the range of situations where women have felt discrimination or insensitivity related to their pregnancy and childbirth experiences. It's important to create a supportive environment that respects each woman's individual journey and to challenge stereotypes or biases that contribute to feelings of discrimination.

Now, the question is, why C-sec rate is increasing in India? There is an article that suggests

https://www.ncbi.nlm.nih.gov/pmc/articles/PMC8797113/

- C-section deliveries are more prevalent in South Indian states compared to North Indian states. Additionally, these kinds of deliveries are performed more frequently in urban areas than in rural areas.
- Literacy and the increasing age at which women give birth play an important role in C-section deliveries. They are directly proportional to the increasing rate of C-section deliveries.
- Private institutions are performing more C-section deliveries than public health institutions. This is associated with women belonging to the upper-middle class and wealthy households who mostly opt for deliveries in private institutions due to a perception of better service provision and higher quality of care.
- Spreading awareness about the importance of normal delivery when no medical complications are present in women is important. This can be achieved through

primary care providers and frontline workers who are often the first point of contact for pregnant women for ANC care, routine check-ups, and visits related to any pregnancy complications.

Changes in C-section deliveries across the Indian states, NFHS (2015-2020)

States/UTs	NFHS-4 (2015-2016)	NFHS-5 (2019-2020)	AC	RC
Lakshadweep	38.4	31.3	-7.1	-18.5
Mizoram	12.7	10.8	-1.9	-15.0
Nagaland	5.8	5.2	-0.6	-10.3
Telangana	57.7	60.7	3.0	5.2
Andhra Pradesh	40.1	42.4	2.3	5.7
Kerala	40.1	42.4	2.3	5.7
Meghalaya	7.6	8.2	0.6	7.9
Gujarat	18.4	21.0	2.6	14.1
Manipur	21.1	25.6	4.5	21.3
Tripura	20.5	25.1	4.6	22.4
Jammu and Kashmir	33.4	41.7	8.3	24.9
Himachal Pradesh	16.7	21.0	4.3	25.7
Goa	31.4	39.5	8.1	25.8

States/UTs	NFHS-4 (2015-2016)	NFHS-5 (2019-2020)	AC	RC
Maharashtra	20.1	25.4	5.3	26.4
Karnataka	23.6	31.5	7.9	33.5
Assam	13.4	18.1	4.7	35.1
West Bengal	23.8	32.6	8.8	37.0
Dadra and Nagar Haveli and Daman and Diu	16.1	22.9	6.8	42.2
Andaman and Nicobar	19.3	29.9	10.6	54.9
Bihar	6.2	9.7	3.5	56.5
Sikkim	20.9	32.8	11.9	56.9
Ladakh	16.1	37.6	21.5	133.5

AC: Absolute change, RC: Relative change

The c-section rate in India has been steadily increasing over the years. According to the National Family Health Survey (NFHS) conducted in 2015-2016, the c-section rate in India was approximately 17.2%. However, it's important to note that c-section rates can vary significantly between different states and regions within the country. The Indian government has been actively monitoring and addressing the rising c-section rates, as it has become a matter of concern for public health. Efforts are being made to promote natural childbirth and ensure that c-sections are only performed when medically necessary for the well-being of the mother and the baby.

As an author, regardless of the type of delivery, every mother's experience is unique and valid. It's crucial to promote a supportive and non-judgmental environment where mothers are celebrated for their strength, resilience, and love for their children. Your message can help create awareness and understanding, fostering a sense of unity among mothers and encouraging empathy and compassion towards all childbirth experiences.

CHAPTER 9

POSTPARTUM AND HEALING

As Beena cradles her one-month-old baby, she feels a wave of overwhelming fatigue wash over her. The sleepless nights and the constant demands of motherhood have taken a toll on her, both physically and emotionally. She has to wake up at unknown times in the night to feed her baby and clean her up while he pees. She gazes down at her precious bundle of joy, feeling a mix of love and vulnerability, but also the weight of the immense responsibility that comes with being a new mother.

One day she picked her up and unknowingly said, "Ravi, can you please pass the diaper bag?"

"It is right next to your left hand, and I am at a 10 ft distance from you," replied Ravi.

"But I am holding the baby too along with the poop, this will spread everywhere if I leave her," replied Beena.

"You have all day to sleep and take care of the baby during your maternity leave. Still, you expect me to keep helping you after my troubled office hours. Here you go, take it," Ravi replied, handing over the diaper bag to Beena.

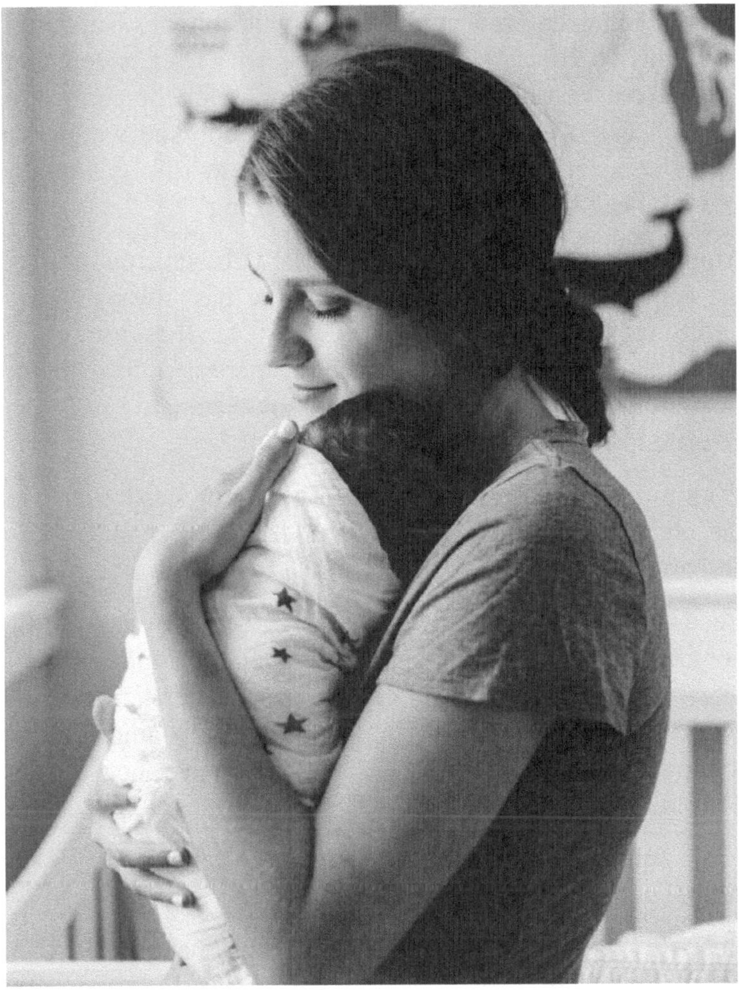

"She is not only my baby. She is your responsibility too, and you must understand, I can't even sleep during the day. I feed her every 3 hours; she is just 20 days old. Don't you have any attachment to the baby? Why do I wake up at night alone?" Beena replied in a stern tone.

Ravi shrugged off her voice and went to sit on the sofa next to him.

Ravi remained preoccupied with his phone, seemingly oblivious to Beena's struggle. The distance between them feels like a vast chasm, and Beena longs for the connection they once shared before the baby arrived. She wonders if Ravi understands the magnitude of her new role as a mother and if he can see the challenges she's facing.

Anita, Beena's mother-in-law, stands with her arms crossed, her face etched with disapproval. She has always been a traditional woman, adhering strictly to the norms and expectations of society. In her mind, there is a clear picture of what a perfect wife and mother should be, and she doesn't hesitate to vocalize her criticisms.

With a disapproving tone, Anita said, "You can't even feed the child on time, Beena. No wonder he's become such a crybaby!"

Beena's heart sinks with each word, her own insecurities heightened by the judgmental words of her mother-in-law. She knows that her baby's crying is not a reflection of her abilities as a mother, but the criticism only amplifies her feelings of inadequacy. Beena thought in her head, "Why don't you ask your son to help?"

Anita continued, "And look at her! She's gone so weak. You should be taking better care of her."

Beena's eyes welled up with tears, but she blinked them away, unwilling to show weakness in front of Anita. She has been trying her best to care for her baby, but the constant comments about her perceived shortcomings made her feel like she is failing at motherhood.

Meanwhile, Ravi finally glanced up from his phone, but his eyes seemed distant, and his mind still elsewhere. He is torn between the love he has for his wife and child and the expectation of being a dutiful son, caught in the middle of his mother's disapproval and Beena's struggle.

Anita pointed out more faults, "You haven't given her the medicines on time either. What kind of mother are you?"

Beena's throat tightened, and she fought to hold back the tears that threatened to spill over. She feels like she is drowning in a sea of expectations, struggling to keep her head above the water. The weight of being a new mother, combined with the constant criticism, has pushed her into a state of despair.

Beena replied softly, "I'm trying my best, Maa. It's just overwhelming, and I need some support either from you or from Ravi."

Anita, who remained unmoved, said, "Support? You should know how to take care of your child. You can't even do simple things like clipping her nails or bathing her properly, leave aside cleaning her poop."

Beena's heart breaks a little more with each hurtful word.

Beena replied, "I know I am still learning, and the journey of motherhood is filled with challenges, but the criticism from you makes me feel like I am a failure. I long for understanding and empathy, but it seems like an impossible dream from mother and son."

Beena further added, struggling to hold back tears, "Maybe I need some time to figure things out. I'll go stay with my parents for a while. Maybe there, I can find some mental peace."

Without waiting for a response, Beena gently places her baby in the pram, gathers a few essentials, and leaves the room. Ravi finally looks up, realizing the gravity of the situation.

Ravi: (calling out) Beena, wait!

But Beena doesn't stop. She walks out of the house, her heart heavy with sadness and relief at the same time. The weight of Anita's expectations had become too much to bear, and she knew she needed a break to gather herself and find strength.

Days pass, and Beena finds solace in her parents' house. They welcome her with open arms, offering comfort and understanding without judgment. As she spends time with her baby in the serene atmosphere of her childhood home, Beena begins to find the strength to confront her postpartum depression and regain her sense of self.

The support from her parents helps Beena realize that being a mother is not about perfection or meeting societal expectations. It's about unconditional love, patience, and learning from the challenges that come with motherhood. As she starts to heal, Beena also reflects on her relationship with Ravi. She longs for open communication and shared responsibilities, hoping that they can grow together as a family.

Back at her in-law's house, Ravi and Anita begin to recognize the impact of their words and actions. The absence of Beena and the baby leaves a void, one that can't be filled with criticism and blame. In time, Beena returns to her home, but with a newfound sense of strength and determination. She sits down with Ravi and Anita, laying bare her feelings and struggles. They have difficult conversations, but with each word spoken, a path to healing and understanding begins to emerge.

Beena adds firmly, "I need your support, Ravi. Being a mother is not easy, and I can't do it alone. Let's learn together and be there for each other and our baby. I need support from Maa as well. Constructive criticism is fine, but calling me out for everything that goes bad is really unfair."

Ravi listens, his heart heavy with guilt for not being more supportive earlier. He realizes that being a partner means being present in both the joys and challenges of parenthood.

A woman's journey through postpartum depression is not easy, but with the love and support of her husband and her in-laws, she learns to manage it better. She becomes more confident as a mother, embracing the imperfections and finding joy in the little moments. Together, the family creates a nurturing environment for the baby, one filled with love, understanding, and acceptance. The weight of societal expectations gradually fades, replaced by a genuine connection between them all.

In time, the scars from the past begin to heal, and the family moves forward with renewed hope and a shared commitment to supporting each other through life's challenges. The journey isn't perfect, but they learn that the strength of their bond lies in their willingness to grow and learn together as a family.

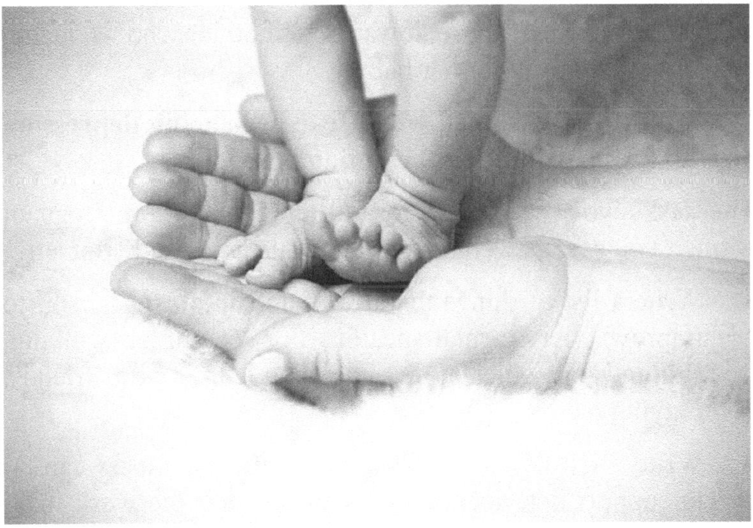

What can you do to support the woman at your home?

The article from *https://www.ncbi.nlm.nih.gov/* talks about

how to take care of the postpartum women.
Women who experience depression during or after childbirth require emotional support. Assure them that this condition is often temporary and can affect some women who have recently given birth. It can be helpful for women to understand that feeling depressed after the birth of a baby is a normal occurrence, and many women go through similar feelings. It's important to communicate with the woman's family and emphasize the need for additional support during this period. Make sure that both she and the newborn are receiving the necessary care.

In some cases, relatives and even healthcare professionals might not take the concerns of these women seriously. If a woman perceives that her concerns are being dismissed, it can contribute to feelings of inadequacy as a mother, which can worsen her depression. Certain mothers may struggle to care adequately for themselves and their baby. This situation is particularly relevant for women with special needs and, in some cases, adolescents. It's crucial that no one engages in verbal or physical abuse towards a mother who is facing challenges in caring for her baby.

Ways to support women who are experiencing depression or who require additional emotional support.

The tasks you carry out for all the postpartum/pregnant women you see, as well as for your colleagues and yourself!

- Write a list of things that a woman can do for herself to improve her mental health. For example, walking, resting and quiet time, spending time with friends, praying or singing songs.
- Write a list of things that other family members can do to support her, such as helping out with the work load, sitting and listening to her, providing an environment of care and support.

- Create a happy environment at your home and let the postpartum woman feel that this is going to end soon.
- Take extra care of the baby and the mother to ensure that she is not over burdened with the responsibilities.
- Arrange some dinners out of your home, so that she starts to feel normal again.

Conclusion : Who to trust?

A pregnant woman should believe in herself, have faith in God, and trust her doctor. The doctor knows your physical condition and any complications you might have. With experience in dealing with multiple pregnancies, the doctor is equipped to handle issues just like yours.

Author Richa Kumari, who was pregnant, listened to only two voices: a) Her heart, which assured her that everything would be alright, and b) Her doctor Manisha Ranjan, who always provided motivation.

A caring and supportive doctor can greatly inspire pregnant women through clear communication, personalized guidance, and positive reinforcement. Through education, the doctor empowers women with knowledge about the benefits of maintaining an active and healthy lifestyle during pregnancy. Sharing success stories and resources can further inspire them. The doctor's empathy and active listening foster a trusting relationship that helps women address concerns and stay motivated. Ultimately, a good doctor plays a pivotal role in guiding and encouraging pregnant women on their journey towards a healthy pregnancy.

Here, is a small picture of the author with the doctor who supported her through the pregnancy.

Dr. Manisha Ranjan is a Consultant Obstetrician and Gynaecologist with 15 years of experience in these fields. She practices at Nidan Mother and Child Care in Sector-51, Noida, and Aarza Square 2, Greater Noida West. She completed her MBBS from Patliputra Medical College, Dhanbad, in 2001 and her DGO from Rajawadi Hospital Mumbai in 2005. She achieved top honors in her university

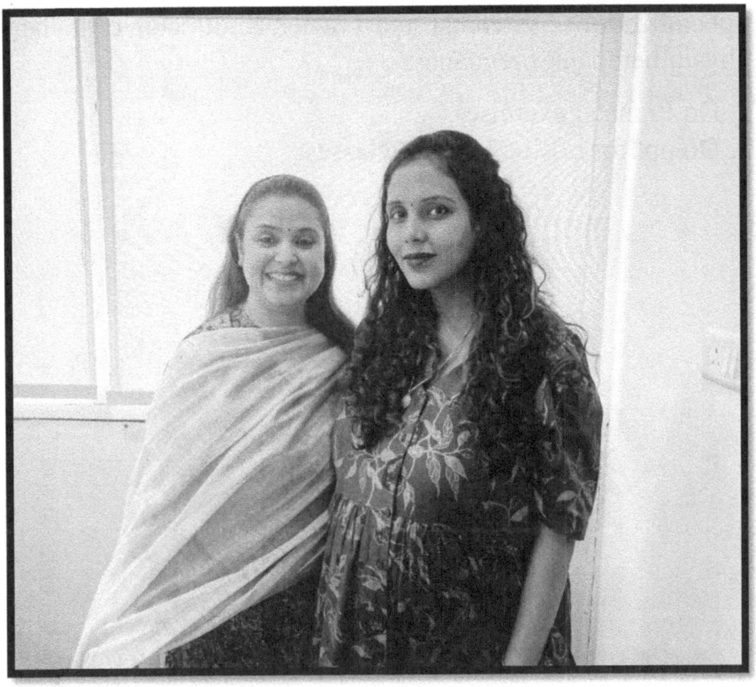

with outstanding results and maintained an exemplary academic record throughout her career. She ranked as the top performer in India for the RSBY project, overseeing more than 7500 cases. She is a member of the Indian Medical Association (IMA) and the Delhi Medical Council. Some of the services provided by the doctor include addressing Gynecological issues, Infertility Evaluation, Delivery, C-section procedures, and Infertility Treatments, among others.

Other things a pregnant women can do keep herself active and positive throughout the pregnancy

1. Join Labour management and Garbh Sanskar Classes. Author joined Dr Reema Ranka's workshops and felt really positive about labour and Delivery.

Dr Reema Ranka (PT), Women's health physiotherapist , Lamaze child birth educator,

Specialization - antenatal and Owner & director of Reborn physiotherapy & pregnancy -

2. Do Prenatal exercises.
3. Do opt for offline Lamaze classes.

Shocking Survey

To claim that the above stated facts in each chapter is not fictious and is being faced by a lot of women these days, Author conducted an anonymous survey on 670 participants (all Pregnant women) .Out of which 78 women responded.

Question 1

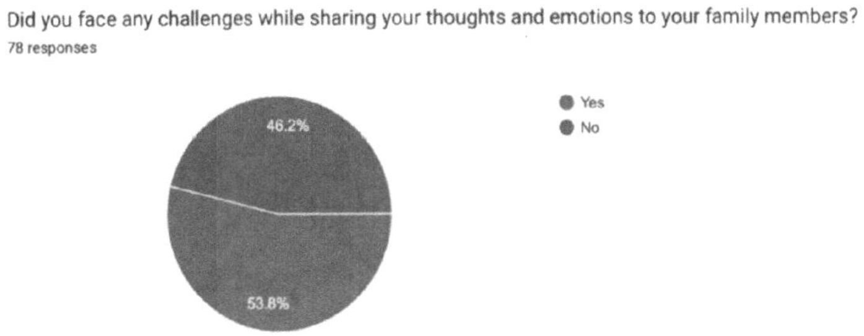

As seen above 53.8% felt challenges sharing their thoughts to their family members.

Question 2

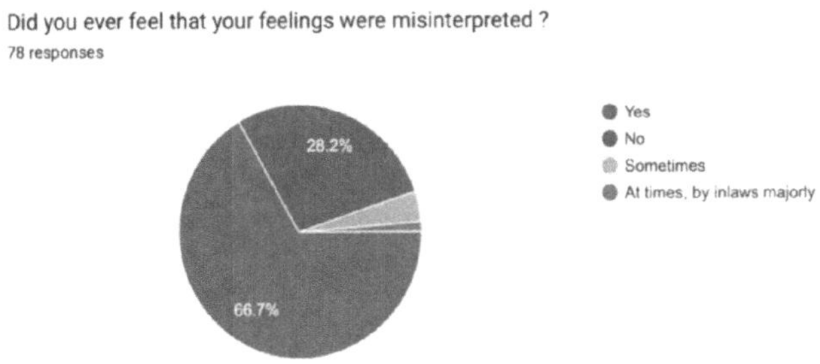

Close to 67% felt that their feelings were misinterpreted. Where are we heading as a family where we can't understand our women?

Question 3

Who was the one person, who caused troubles for you in your pregnancy

78 responses

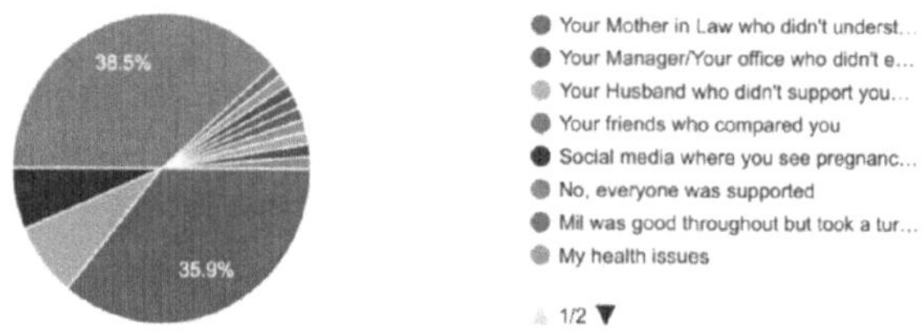

One person who accounted for 35.9% of the trouble for pregnant women was their Mother in law? We claim to be a part of modern civilised society where we treat our daughters and daughter in laws equally. Then, how come we are seeing these numbers? There is something that needs to be changed in the mindset of today's mother in order to reduce the above horrifying numbers.

Similarly, husband needs to be more empathetic by reading more, understanding emotions and learning about pregnancies' complications.

Social Media is also creating troubles and make pregnant women feel less confident about themselves.

But let's not forget about 38.5% data also that reveals everyone was supportive. Thus, we are progressing well and we are about to reach the goal of 100% but it is a long way to go and unless we learn empathy, we won't be able to progress as a society and will end up creating a cage for our pregnant ladies.

Question 4

Author also asked participants to share one statement from the people above or any one incident that hurt the most in women's pregnancy? They were asked to narrate the story :

Participant 1

"MIL not sending me to my home"

Participant 2

"My MIL not allowed me to go to my mother's home, even being in the same city, and wanted me to do all the house hold work as it is good for normal delivery"

Participant 3

"My husband said that you're not the only pregnant woman in the world , people work so much. Never asks me how do I feel"

Participant 4

"Tum akeli nhi ho jo baccha paida kar rhi ho. This is what my MIL said to me whenever i express my feelings. I used to be very protective about my body and health. I knew it that pregnancy is not easy. I got married when I was only 21 yr old. And i used to scared of getting pregnant. Hence somehow I managed to push baby planning till 6yrs of my marriage. To be honest I am still not ready for it neither physically nor mentally. But my forced me to plan a baby..... I am scared of any kind of pain on my body and every person has different level of pain tolerance... whenever I told my in laws that i am having pain or having trouble in doing something they say "sabko baccha hota hai tum akeli nhi ho jo baccha paid karogi" that's hurts a lot".

Participant 5

"Mother in law interference in each and everything. She tries to do things as per her convenience taste and there so called orthodox thinking irritated me a lot".

Participant 6

"My Mother in Law mentally disturbed me".

Participant 7

"Every women deliver, what's a big deal you are overacting!"

Participant 8

"Male colleagues making fun of maternity leave"

Participant 9

"Husband not considering the mood swings I faced".

Participant 10

"I am entering the last week of my pregnancy and my MIL has not asked one once what would I like to eat, or ever cooked or fed me once. She has not asked me any morning that how am I feeling or did I sleep well. Until now in the 33rd week I am cooking for myself and my husband while she feeds and cooks for my FIL and BIL. She never discusses anything or plans anything with me neither how will we do things around delivery time, when and how to pack the hospital bag, nothing at all. Its now SICK and DISGUSTING and FRUSTRATING to even look at her or feel her presence in the same house".

Participant 11

"Everyone was supportive during my pregnancy fortunately. However, I can't say the same during postpartum "

Participant 12

"Created FOMO as I scrolled through social media and other girls of my age enjoying trips and festivals whereas I was on complete bed rest and restricted to home. This created emotional ups and downs for me sometimes in my pregnancy."

Participant 13

"My mil acting as if she was too caring about me ,which is actually not true"

Participant 14

"My Husband didn't understand my feelings".

Participant 15

"I once had severe headache and backache while at a relative's place and informed this to husband and MIL both to take me to home but due to a particular guest we couldn't so I tolerated pain but even when the guest went I was told to corporate just for few minutes then I felt bad that they're not understanding I was pregnant and tolerating isn't easy and incorrect too."

Participant 16

"Frequent misunderstandings of my husband."

Participant 17

"My family called me lazy each time i felt sick in my first trimester and couldnt go for walks as suggested by doc".

Participant 18

"Everyone is supporting me my family, In laws and office staff"

Participant 19

"Superstitious mother-in-law who created toxic environment for me"

Participant 20

"Husband asking to leave job and focus on pregnancy"

Participant 21

"My mother in law made me to do all household chores with heavy works included".

Participant 22

"My husband couldn't handle me. Bcoz mine was over expectation".

Participant 23

"My MIL never came to me for taking my care"

Participant 24

"Mil comparing me with herself that how active she used to be during her time".

Participant 25

"MIL never prepared anything special for me in my entire journey. Infact I used to prepare instead. Hubby sometimes didn't care about my feelings, though most of the times he was supportive & caring. But as they say we remember the negatives more than positives".

Participant 26

"Office workload was the issue"

Participant 27

"My mother-in-law has always been a problem at every phase of my life post marriage".

Participant 28

"Mil is a constant trouble maker. Doesn't help me in my household chores n expects me to do everything being in pain too. She is a toxic lady".

Participant 29

"Loneliness"

Participant 30

"Didn't get that emotional support".

Participant 31

"People forgot who am I and what are my likings/feelings/choices etc and more focused on baby (specially elders who are still following their age old myths which is not at all logical in today's era) which I felt is wrong for a person like me who is more logical, educated and scientific hence doesn't follow everyone's opinion blindly including husband".

Participant 32

"My mother in law not understanding my situation and forcing me to do household work like lifting weights etc"

Participant 33

"I didn't face any of negative situations, all were very supportive".

Participant 34

"Unnecessary arguments with MIL - expected me to handle every households chores. Doctor suggested me not to start walking, not to stand for too long"

Participant 35

"Nothing"

Participant 36

"Mil asked to return their four wheeler when I was in the end of 3rd month inspite of mild SCH bleeding.. so till the end of pregnancy we used only our 2 wheeler and hired cab for all hospital visits".

Participant 37

"MIL always talking about weight gain".

Participant 38

"None as of now"

Participant 39

"Everyone pressuring to be active always".

Participant 40

"To be honest.. I'm blessed with the Best people around me.. I'm working till now, as my due is next week 25th August My husband, family & my office staff is supportive."

Participant 41

"As had a miscarriage before so was told all the negative stuff mostly by the people who by relation are close ones but

I understood they are not that close from now on".

Participant 42

"My mother in law comparing my pregnancy to others".

Participant 43

"My best friends who called me dramatic when I was at the lowest point in my first trimester".

Participant 44

"My mother in law told me not to take afternoon nap even when I was tired because taking nap in afternoon is not something that her family does".

Participant 45

"My mother in law asking me to do the household chores and not appreciating me ever".

Participant 46

"My MIL told me I am working not because of my choice and not because of any need. Her son earns enough to support the family and I working is just a drop in the ocean. So even if I work or doesn't matter. I am giving unwanted attention to my office and neglecting my pregnancy unnecessarily".

Participant 47

"My MIL always asking me to listen to her orthodox advice and eat according to her".

Participant 48

"My husband who was emotionally not accepting the fact that pregnancy is challenging and always remained carefree about it".

Participant 49

"my MIL never supported or cared about my emotions ever. I wish I was with my own family".

Participant 50

"My husband felt that pregnancy is not a disease and it should be considered normal"

Question 5

Author also asked what was the one thing that was missed the most during pregnancy and here are some of the answers

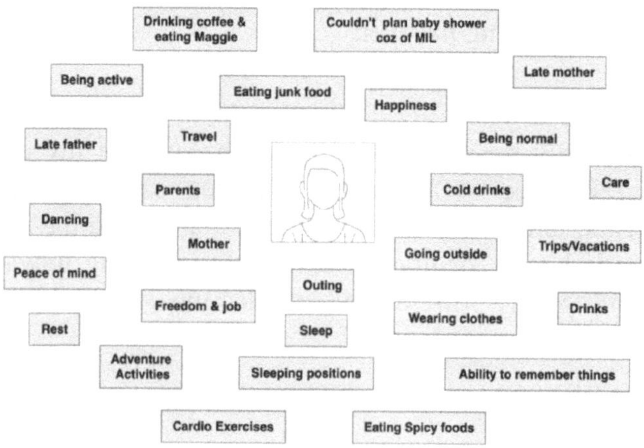

This figure shows that a woman already misses so many things during her pregnancy. On top of that she has following to bear

- Body changes
- Having medicines
- Injections/vaccinations

- Difficulty in passing urine
- Not able to take any medicine, even if ill
- Hormonal changes and mood swings
- Fear of anything going wrong

So, if the woman is already going through so many issues that are physically and emotionally challenging. Isn't it our duty to help our women in the best way possible rather than burdening her with expectations and unnecessary advices.

The Birthing Story

(The birthing story of author's son aims to illustrate what a gentle C-section experience looks like, emphasizing that the role of a positive atmosphere and family support can ensure a smooth and comfortable delivery for women.)

On the evening of August 28th, it was calm, and I had been experiencing regular bowel movements since the morning. I wasn't aware that an upset stomach could be a sign of labor. I sat with my mother on the couch, eagerly awaiting the arrival of my brother and husband so we could enjoy our favorite evening snack, 'Appe.' While sipping on coconut water, I suddenly felt the need to use the restroom. There, I noticed a brown discharge, though I couldn't determine if it was the mucus plug discharge. I made several trips to the bathroom, each time observing the same discharge.

First pregnancies tend to make everyone a bit anxious, and I was no exception. I became slightly nervous and decided to call my doctor. She reassured me that everything was normal and suggested we wait until the pain became unbearable. She advised me to visit her the following day at 7 pm.

I anxiously awaited my husband's return from the office so we could discuss the plan, and I was eager to share the news with my brother as well.

Around 9 pm, my father phoned me and informed me that my brother had to leave Delhi and quickly travel to Mumbai due to unavoidable circumstances. This news hit me hard because my brother had always been there with me through all the ups and downs in life. Even the smallest events in my life had never been without his presence. So, that phone call had a profound impact on me.

When my brother arrived home, he immediately started packing his bags and booking his flight tickets to Mumbai. Our family decided not to mention the discharge, which indicated the onset of labor, until he had secured his tickets. We were concerned that if he found out about it, he might refuse to return to Mumbai. He managed to book the tickets at 11:50 pm, and it was only then that we casually informed him that labor had begun, and we might have the delivery in the next 2-3 days. He became a bit worried, but we assured him that we would manage without him.

Throughout the night, I experienced cramps similar to period pains and couldn't sleep. I was feeling a mix of emotions - happiness because I felt that the time for delivery was approaching, anxiety about the delivery process, and sadness because my brother had left. However, I had the support of my parents and husband.

On the 29th, I woke up in the morning with some soreness near the vagina and a different kind of back pain. I shared with my mother that I had a gut feeling that I might deliver in a day or two. My mother reassured me, saying that whether delivery happened today, tomorrow, or a week from now, it wouldn't matter because I was already 37 weeks and 6 days pregnant, which meant it would be a term baby, and the delivery would not affect the baby.

We began packing our bags, creating two separate bags – one for the baby and another for myself. For the baby, we included items like the lifecell storage bag, a baby's towel, and some clothes. My bag contained items such as maternity pads, a hot water bag, a homecoming outfit, breast pads, maternity bras, and breast cream. The list was quite extensive. This process took about 2 hours, as we had already prepared many of these items during the 34th week of pregnancy.

The car was parked outside, and the clouds hung in the sky. I observed from my balcony, my heart racing with anticipation. Our appointment with the doctor was scheduled for 6 pm, and we aimed to depart while there was still daylight to avoid any last-minute rush. My brother called to inquire about my well-being, and I couldn't express how much I missed him.

My mother lovingly fed me yogurt and sugar, offering her prayers and applying a tiny kumkum mark from the deity's feet. We were prepared for the most significant day of our lives, marking the bittersweet conclusion of a nine-month journey.

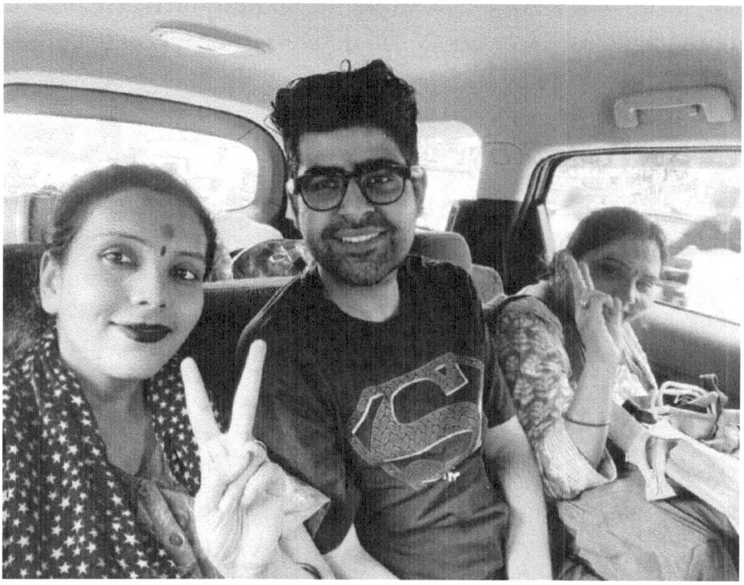

We anxiously awaited the moment to meet our baby, and my mom reassured me, saying, "Relax, dear, everything will be fine. Just remember that you've completed nine months, and this will be a matter of nine hours." We arrived at the doctor's clinic around 6:04 pm and inquired about our appointment. The receptionist informed us, "Ma'am has gone to the hospital (Motherhood Hospital) for an emergency C-section and will return by 7 pm."

We waited in a beautifully decorated hall spanning about 1800 square feet, reciting mantras. We didn't know if today would be the day for my delivery or if it would happen in two days, but we had a strong sense that things were falling into place.

Finally, at 7:29 pm, our doctor arrived. My mom, dad, and husband accompanied me into the room, and the doctor greeted us with a smile. "Richa, lie down. We'll perform a membrane sweep, and you'll need to be admitted to the hospital today. Speak to Jyoti for room booking," the doctor said. I was trembling, as I knew my time was near, but I felt a sense of joy knowing that my baby would soon be in my arms.

The doctor performed the sweep, which, to be honest, was excruciatingly painful for me. Some people barely feel it, but for others, like me, it was painful. It felt like period cramps in my back and a rough, scratching sensation. I tried not to scream, but I couldn't help it.

"You'll worry my other patients waiting outside," the doctor said in a cheerful tone. "Okay, dear, you can now proceed to the hospital, and they will initiate all the necessary processes. Best of luck, dear."

Returning to my 32nd week of pregnancy, my baby had a single loop of the umbilical cord around his neck, and his weight was in the 75th percentile. This situation persisted until the 36th week, with the cord loop not resolving. Being a first-time pregnant woman, even the slightest issues became causes for concern. For me, this was a point of worry, especially because I had always hoped for a normal delivery. I was a bit apprehensive about the possibility of needing a C-section. Additionally, during the 37th-week scan, it was revealed that the baby's weight had reached 3.6 kg, which was on the higher side. Both of these complications had been present since the 32nd week.

Fast forward to August 29th at 8 pm, the doctor had assured me that we would aim for a normal delivery if everything progressed well, regardless of the cord and the baby's weight, citing past successful cases. This boosted my confidence, and I eagerly headed to the hospital.

While in the car, I contacted Jyoti, the counselor at Motherhood, and booked my room. The room, located on the 2nd floor, was a beautifully decorated suite. It consisted of an initial room with a large table, two chairs, and a TV. Inside, there was a patient room with another TV and an attached washroom equipped with a shower and accessories. It was very comfortable and even had a sofa near the bed for someone to sleep on.

On August 29th, at 8:55 pm, I was instructed to change into hospital attire, and a tag with my admission time, name, and blood group was affixed to my right hand. To be honest, I was quite scared about what would happen next. I was unfamiliar with the procedures and had no idea how long my delivery would take.

Soon, a nurse wearing a pink gown arrived with a tray in hand. She entered, drew curtains around my bed, and inserted a cannula into my left hand, limiting my mobility. Then, there was another knock, and a shorter lady in a black co-ord outfit, who didn't seem like a nurse but had a tray, entered. She placed a trimmer nearby and attached a new blade to it. She then pulled the curtain and prepared the area below.

We had opted for a package from the hospital that included various amenities, such as medical supplies, baby vaccinations, photography, room and car decoration, cake cutting, and, of course, complimentary meals (one for the family and always for the patient). Around 9:30 pm, my dinner arrived, consisting of a light meal of Daliya andKhichdi, which I enjoyed wholeheartedly. I decided to start walking as recommended by the workshops I had attended, including Healing Sutras, Reema Ranka's classes, and the Lamaze session by Dr. Sonia Verma. As I contemplated getting up from my bed, a duty doctor arrived along with the nurse. It was quite an intimidating moment because I knew that this was the exact time when my medical procedures would commence. The duty doctor began to tell me the procedure.

"So, we will perform a pelvic exam and apply a gel to soften the cervix. Then, at 5 am, we'll use another gel to further dilate the cervix. We'll repeat this process until 10 am and assess the extent of cervical dilation," explained the doctor. After conducting a cervical examination, she mentioned that my cervix was only 1 cm dilated and proceeded to apply the first round of gel. The pelvic exam was painless, and the gel was inserted gently.

Subsequently, the nurse informed me that they would need to conduct NST (Non-Stress Test) exams after each gel application to monitor the baby's well-being and the adequacy of my contractions. The monitor began beeping, and I noticed my contractions ranging from 0 to 132. I started experiencing contractions every 2 minutes, but to be honest, they weren't too painful.

My father and I began reminiscing about our school memories, discussing how I used to play on the school campus and was known as one of the mischievous children. The pain continued until 3 pm, and suddenly, I felt a reduction in pain, so I tried to get some sleep. However, I couldn't fall asleep, so my husband suggested we take a walk. We strolled along the corridor, which was vibrant with colorful decorations. Outside each room, there were blue or pink balloons, creating a refreshing and comforting atmosphere. We walked until 3:40 am and then decided to rest. It was the most anxious nap of my life, and I couldn't help but watch the clock, which was about to strike 5 am.

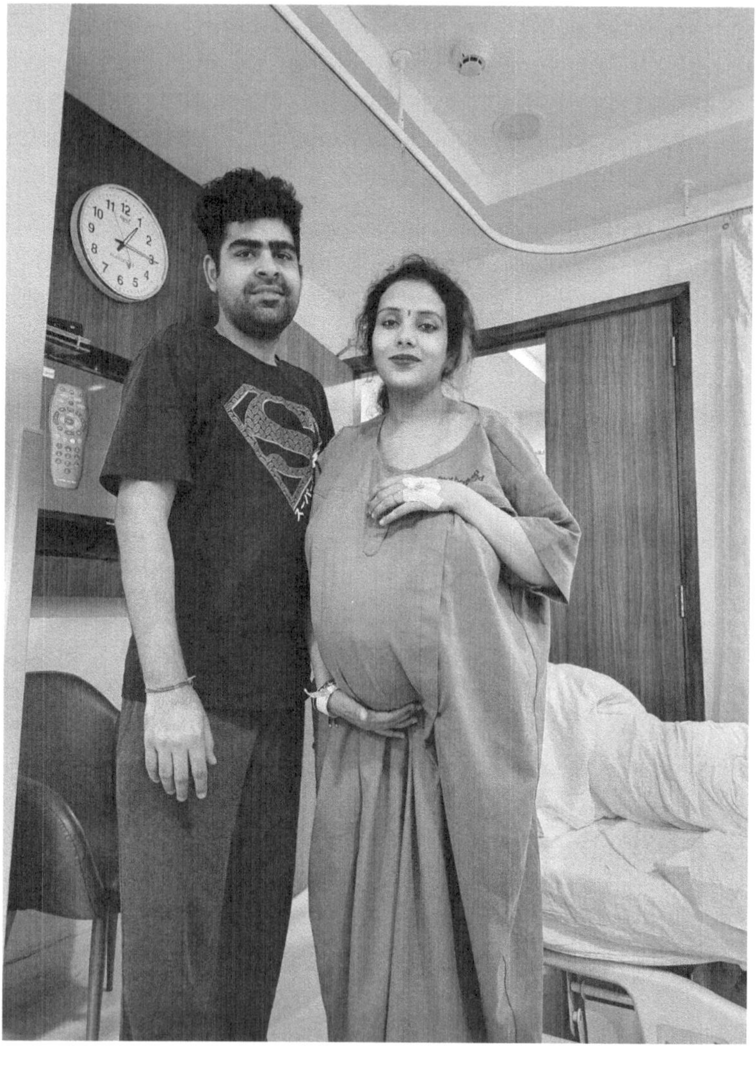

I was awakened by a sudden knock on the door, and it was the same duty doctor who had applied the gel at 10 pm the previous night. She had come with the nurse, who had the pelvic examination tray.

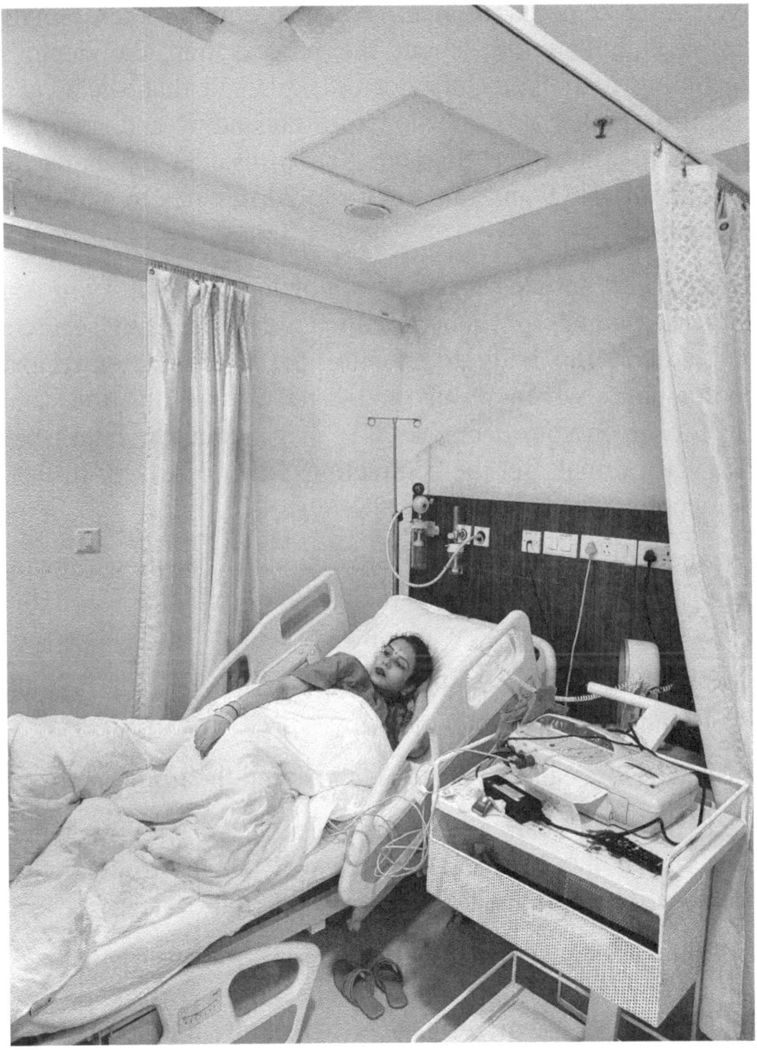

This time, I was hopeful that my cervix would have dilated to 5 cm, and I would soon have a normal delivery, especially after hearing about a friend who had a similar experience. To my surprise, my cervix was only 1.5 cm dilated. I wondered what had happened throughout the night. I had tried squats, walks, and various techniques, but my cervix hadn't dilated even after 6 hours of pain. I was becoming increasingly stressed and anxious about the process and the doctor's upcoming plan. The duty doctor explained that she would perform another gel insertion (prostaglandin) and return at 10 am to assess the dilation. She instructed the nurse to conduct the NST and then return in 20 minutes to apply the gel again.

The NST is perhaps the most annoying procedure you can subject a woman to when she's already in pain. They secure a belt around the belly to monitor the fetal heart rate and contractions, which means you can't change positions and have to lie on your back. My NST began, and the fetal heart rate was normal, but the contractions had decreased. In fact, the score was only around 9-10.

I said to my husband, "Maybe the medications aren't having an effect on me because I'm ahead of schedule, and the artificial induction isn't working as expected."

My husband, Tarun, replied, "Just be patient; it will dilate. By 12 pm, we'll welcome our baby."

I asked, "How can you be so certain about the timing?"

He explained, "Normally, labor doesn't exceed 15-16 hours. That's what I've heard. Only time will tell the truth. If that holds, we should have the baby by 1 pm at the latest."

After the NST, the doctor arrived. She was dressed in a black salwar kameez and had rather large, pretty eyes. She had applied mascara, which enhanced her beauty, but I joked that whatever she was about to do wouldn't be beautiful in any sense. She reapplied the gel, which wasn't painful at all, and she asked, "Now that the cervix has softened, the dilation will begin."

I was filled with happiness at that moment because I had a strong conviction that the situation would improve, and I would be dilated within a few hours, leading to a normal delivery. To manage the pain, I attempted breathing exercises and ball exercises, but unfortunately, the ball exercises exacerbated my discomfort. The only relief came from walking.

Following the gel insertion, another NST was conducted. Additionally, after the gel was applied, it was recommended not to get up for at least 20 minutes. So, despite the pain, I endured it while lying down to allow the gel to take effect and the NST to be completed.

At 8 am, my breakfast was served – idli and sambhar. However, I refrained from eating it entirely, fearing the possibility of an emergency C-section. I wanted to keep my bowels empty.

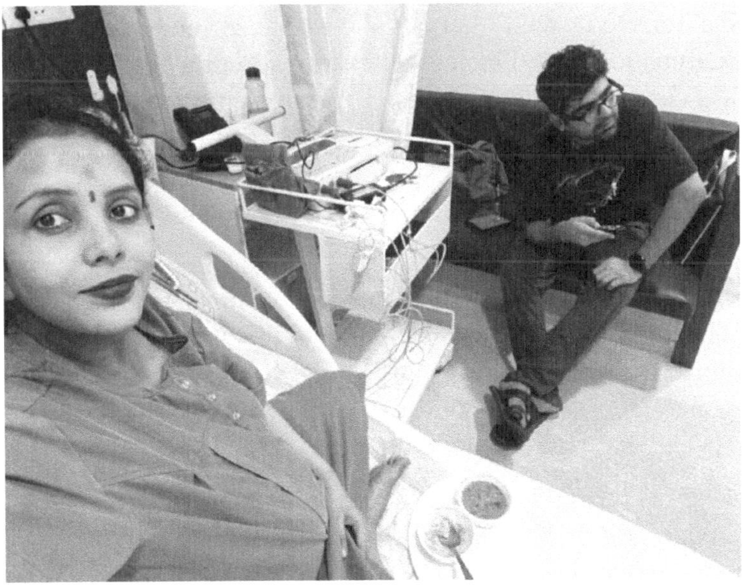

Time seemed to pass incredibly slowly; every second felt like an hour, and every hour like a year. The pain had intensified significantly, making me feel somewhat disoriented. I prayed continuously for my cervix to dilate. My father assisted me in walking along the corridor, while my mother and husband placed a hot water bag on my back. Additionally, due to the baby's weight, my right pelvis had been causing severe pain, making walking difficult for several days. Consequently, my pace was slow and subdued. I intermittently drank water to distract myself from the pain and stay hydrated.

After what felt like an eternity, the clock finally struck ten, and I entered the room, eagerly awaiting the doctor's arrival to check the dilation progress. I heard a knock on the door, and the morning shift nurse arrived. She was slightly overweight and wore the same pink uniform, appearing to be around 40 years old. Her demeanor seemed a bit intimidating, and her assertive voice heightened my anxiety because I wasn't certain if the pain would continue to prolong.

She arrived with her NST machine and the pelvic examination tray. Placing the examination tray at the bottom of a cart, she initiated the NST to assess the fetal well-being before applying the third gel. The contractions reached a score of 128-135, and the fetal heart rate remained within the normal range.

The nurse likely informed the duty doctor, who returned after 20 minutes to conduct another examination. She stated, "The dilation is only 2 cm so far, and this is the last gel I will apply. We can't keep using gel. Let me perform the sweep again."

I began shouting and screaming at the top of my lungs because I couldn't endure the rough membrane sweep. Anxiety overwhelmed me as it seemed my body wasn't cooperating.

Then, my doctor, Manisha ma'am, arrived and learned that it had been 12 hours without any cervical dilation. She instructed the nurse, saying, "Keep her under monitoring, and I will return at 1 pm to assess the cervix. If she's dilated by then, great; otherwise, we'll assess the situation."

The doctor left, and my mother and my husband (TARUN) followed her to inquire about what she meant by "the situation" and if there were any risks involved.

My mom returned and said, "She will return at 1 pm and then decide on the next steps. She asked us not to panic and to support you during this time."

I can confirm that from 10 am to 1:30 pm on August 30th, it was the most excruciating pain I had ever experienced in my life. I couldn't focus on anything. I just practiced breathing exercises and kept walking to pass the time. It was a dreadful and traumatizing experience, with cervical checks every two hours causing pain. Simultaneously, contractions continued, and NST tests were conducted repeatedly.

Finally, it was 1 pm, and I was relieved that it was time for Manisha ma'am to return. I had an inexplicable trust in her. She arrived around 1:10 pm, and I was in excruciating pain. She instructed the nurse who accompanied her to bring the pelvic examination kit. I had a strong feeling that she would perform a membrane sweep, and my gut feeling proved correct. Alongside the contractions I was already enduring, she performed the membrane sweep, which was unbearable. I started screaming in frustration and asked her to stop. My husband yelled from behind, "Go ahead with it; otherwise, you might face extended labor."

I decided to relax a bit and allowed the doctor to perform the sweep. By that point, it was becoming clear to me that the gels and medications weren't having the desired effect on my body. I was becoming increasingly stressed and anxious about what would come next.

The combination of the membrane sweep, contractions, and the NST belt had made the overall situation quite traumatizing for me. The doctor then informed me, "You are only dilated to 2.75 to 3 cm, and this is going to be a challenging journey since dilation is progressing slowly. If the pain becomes unbearable, we can offer you an epidural."

I nodded in agreement, as I was in excruciating pain and significant discomfort. The doctor instructed the nurse, saying, "Administer some medication along with the IV, and if the pain remains unbearable, we will provide the epidural around 2 pm."

At 2 pm, a stretcher arrived to transport me. I had always thought that an epidural was just an injection, but it turned out to involve the insertion of a tiny catheter at the top of the spine, with the epidural then being administered to alleviate the pain. However, I wasn't aware of this and had assumed I would mostly be taken to a triage room where my husband would be with me.

But life doesn't always go as planned; it's often in the hands of fate. I was taken to the operating room (OT) because that's where epidurals are administered. I began to cry, pleading with them to allow my husband inside, as I believed that with his presence, I could manage everything more peacefully. Unfortunately, the nurses did not permit him to enter the OT.

Then another nurse arrived and asked me to undergo a cervical check. I told her that I didn't want to be checked again, as I had been examined just at 1 pm and was already 2.5-3 cm dilated, experiencing severe pain.

The nurse agreed and said, "Alright, we won't perform the sweep, and we won't do the pelvic examination. Just relax for now, and let's proceed to the OT for the epidural."

"So my husband can't accompany me?" I inquired.

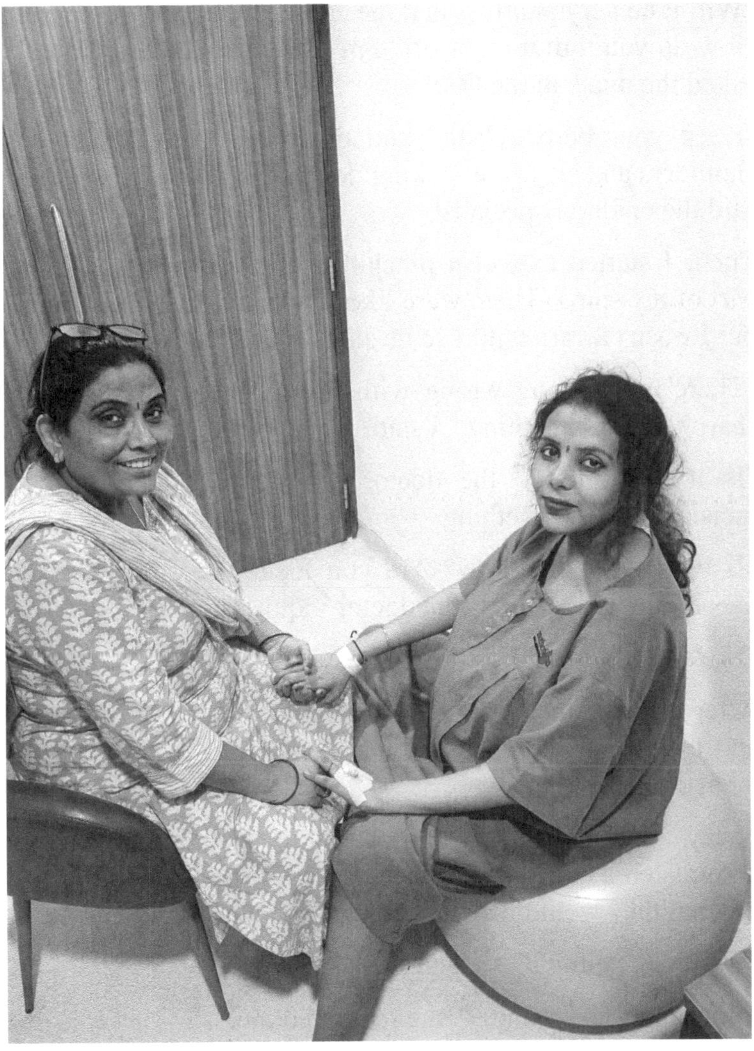

"No, ma'am, it's against the rules, and we won't be able to allow that at any point," she responded.

Finally, I was taken to the OT for the epidural, and the room was quite cold. I was shivering when the doctor arrived to administer the epidural.

"Will it be very painful? Is it the catheter that will be inserted? How do you turn it on or off? I'm really scared," I repeatedly asked the nurse in the OT.

"Keep your body relaxed and don't tense up. Relax your shoulders and sit while looking down. We're about to begin," said the epidural specialist.

Then, I started to feel a pinching sensation near the lower part of my spine. There were likely two incisions being made, but I wasn't aware until I felt a sharp jolt in my right leg.

"There's something wrong with my right leg; it felt like a sharp jerk or something," I said.

"Is it okay now?" the doctor asked while adjusting the incision site or something.

"Is everything fine now? Are you feeling any pain in your legs or anywhere else?" the doctor inquired.

"No, sir, nothing at all," I replied.

After that, the incision site was taped to secure the epidural, and I was transferred to another stretcher to be taken to the labor room.

I lay silently in the labor room with the epidural administered in my back. Then, a nurse arrived and informed me that they would insert a catheter and attach a urine bag.

"Will it be painful?" I asked.

"You won't feel a thing," she reassured me.

"But it did feel tight down there when they inserted the catheter. Then, the day shift doctor arrived after 15 minutes to perform a cervical examination. She asked me to move, but I couldn't because my right leg was completely numb, and I couldn't even move it an inch. The epidural doctor was called to double-check if the epidural was properly placed. Meanwhile, the doctor began the cervical examination, and I was only dilated to about 2.5-3 cm.

She said, 'No one else will perform the pelvic exam except me, and I'll return to check on it by 5 pm. It was exactly 3 pm at that moment. The NST belt was strapped over my belly, the BP machine was monitoring my blood pressure, and an oxygen mask was provided to assist with my breathing.

Suddenly, I heard my husband's voice, and I felt elated. Then, my mother entered the room as well. I became more confident that things would work out. I hoped that within the next two hours, I would dilate further and perhaps have a normal delivery.

I then drifted off to sleep, a deep sleep, as if I hadn't been awakened the entire previous night. I could see nurses coming in and adding some medications to my IV from time to time. They checked for contractions and monitored the fetal heartbeat.

I didn't realize when the clock struck 5 pm. Ideally, I should have seen some progress in terms of dilation. After all, it had been 21 hours of labor.

I could see my husband waiting to perform the pelvic examination and inform us about the progress of dilation. He came and called Manisha Ranjana while conducting the examination. 'Ma'am, it's still 3 cm, and the baby's head hasn't descended much. It's in a mid-position, pp-2,' said the day shift doctor to Manisha ma'am over the phone.

'Add some medication and give her a tablet to place under her tongue,' instructed Manisha ma'am, which the nurse did. I didn't quite understand what was happening, and I began to lose confidence that I would have a normal delivery.

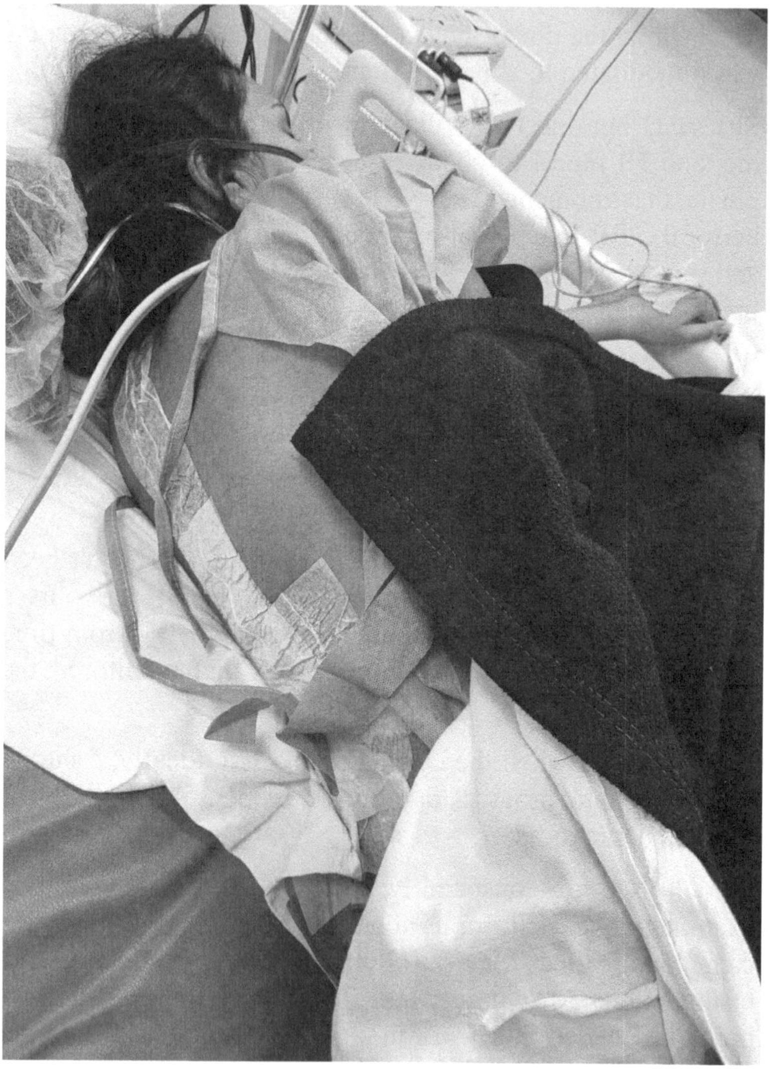

Other nurses and staff at the hospital mentioned that they had seen cases where dilation occurred after 36 hours, and for now, the situation was under control. The amniotic sac hadn't ruptured, the baby wasn't in distress, and the mother was fine. As a result, we could wait for the cervix to dilate and opt for a vaginal delivery.

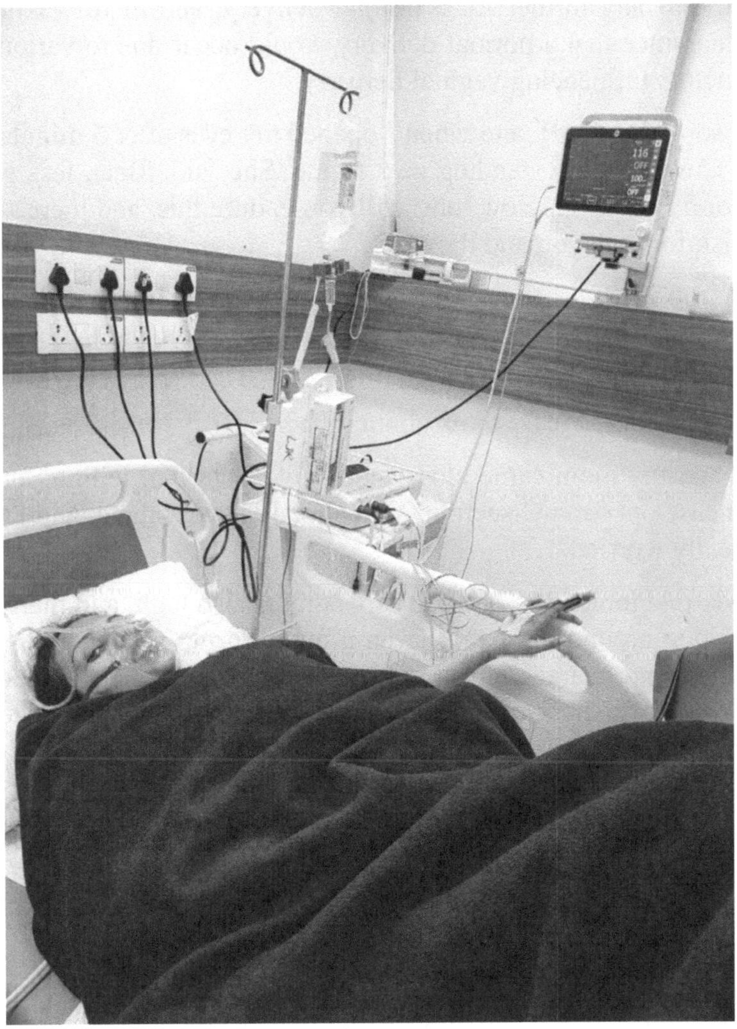

My husband asked, 'So, we don't know when it will dilate, and we don't know when the delivery will happen, right?'

'Yes, sir, we have no idea about that part,' replied the staff.

My husband stepped outside to speak with my parents. He was very concerned because he didn't want me to push myself any further for a normal delivery, and there was no guarantee that a normal delivery would occur due to various factors influencing vaginal delivery.

I soon dozed off, and when I opened my eyes after 5 minutes, I saw my mom standing next to me. She said, 'Beta, let's go for a C-section. How long will you endure this, and there's a risk for both you and the baby.'

Tarun (my husband) chimed in, 'Yeah, Richa, I agree. Please consider it, as the delay may pose a risk to you and the baby, and we can't afford that.'

'I'll be back. Please think about it,' he added.

Then my mom came closer and said, 'Beta, I'm telling you, please opt for a C-section. You already have asthma, and I'm really worried.'

My dad joined in, 'The baby's weight is also high, and there's a loop around the baby. Even after enduring so much pain, there's no guarantee of a normal delivery. The medical team is doing their best, but luck is unpredictable. So, it's better not to wait for uncertainty.'

I wasn't initially convinced, but then I glanced at my parents, and suddenly, a quote from the movie K3G came to mind where Shahrukh Khan says, "In life, if you want to achieve something, if you want to attain something, listen to your heart. And if even your heart doesn't have an answer, close your eyes and take your parents' names. You will overcome every difficulty; every destination will be yours, just yours."

(,"zindagi me agar Kuch jeetna ho Kuch hassil karna ho to apne dil ki suno aur agar dil b koi jawab na de ro aankhein band kar apne mummy papa ka naam lo, Tum har mushkil par kar jaoge , har manzil Tumhari hogi, Sirf Tumhari")

In that very moment, I decided to trust my parents and my husband's instincts and went along with what they suggested. I agreed to the surgery. My mother called my doctor and requested a C-section. It had already been 21 hours, and my family was growing anxious about the delivery.

In the labor room, the nurse received the call from the doctor, and everything around me began to change. The nurse who had been caring for me asked me to discard the tablet I had been given to place under my tongue. She informed me that Manisha ma'am would arrivc in 10 minutes for the C-section.

The epidural was turned off, and the other nurses inquired, "Should we administer enigma? When did you last eat?"

"Around 12 pm, and it was a very light meal," I replied.

"Lct's move her to the operating room now."

I could hear their voices, and I was filled with fear because everything was happening so quickly, and I wasn't mentally prepared for it at all.

As I was being transported to the operating room, I could see my parents and husband appearing nervous. Their smiles seemed forced, and I could sense their anxiety. I closed my eyes and put my trust in God.

Inside the operating room, the anesthetist and a team of nurses were waiting. The room was quite cold, and I was moved onto the sleek operating table. The anesthetist instructed me to look down, removed the epidural, and informed me that he would administer medication to numb my lower body for the surgery.

Then, I heard the comforting voice of my lucky charm, Manisha ma'am. She gazed at me, and I returned her gaze as she encouraged me to smile. She asked, "Richa, what's your favorite song?" and mentioned that she would play it. At first, I thought she was joking, but she asked again.

I replied, " 'Badtameez Dil'."

She played the song, instantly lightening the mood in the operating room. Manisha ma'am came closer and said, "Your child is special, this bed is lucky, the day is lucky, and the number is lucky." I didn't fully understand her words, but I assumed she was trying to boost my morale.

Then, with the anesthetist's assistance, I gradually lost sensation in the catheter and the pain in my leg subsided. I couldn't feel anything in the lower part of my body.

I glanced at the set of scissors nearby, realizing the multitude of instruments used in surgeries. It was a somewhat eerie feeling.

Everything was prepared, and it was time for the surgery. I was instructed to lie down, and various monitors like the BP machine, ECG, and oximeter were attached to me. There was an IV drip, the contents of which I was unaware of. A curtain was placed in front of me, obscuring my view and sensations.

My anesthetist proved to be an incredibly supportive presence. He engaged in conversation with me, asking about my history of asthma, where I lived, and my parents' residence. His soothing interaction helped me remain calm during those crucial minutes.

In precisely five minutes, I heard a baby cry, and the doctor exclaimed, "It's a chubby baby!"

I couldn't comprehend that it was my baby crying because it had only been five minutes, and I couldn't fathom how a child could arrive so quickly.

Suddenly, everyone in the room erupted into applause, and there was a celebratory atmosphere. Some people from outside the operating room entered, and there was a flurry of picture-taking. I longed to catch a glimpse of my child, but I could hear that there was still activity happening on my abdomen.

I assumed this might be a routine part of every delivery, unaware that this delivery was extraordinary, my baby was extraordinary, and my doctor was extraordinary.

Then, everything started to change.

A nurse approached me and revealed my baby to me. It was a moment of love at first sight, and I couldn't hold back my tears. I could see those tiny feet and fingers. All I could think was that I had brought this little human into the world. I didn't care whether it was a boy or a girl; it was my baby, and that was all that mattered. The nurse gently placed the baby's skin against mine, and I cried once more. She asked me to guess the gender, and suddenly, she revealed that it was a boy. My precious baby had arrived at 6:21 pm on August 30th. I couldn't hold back my tears once more, and I could feel the stitches on my abdomen. It felt like a tap on my stomach, and I realized it would be a permanent scar, a reminder of my accomplishment.

It no longer mattered whether it was a C-section or a natural delivery. All that mattered was that my baby was healthy.

The doctor informed me that he weighed 3.9 kilograms and then took him for a bath.

I eagerly awaited the arrival of my mom, dad, and Tarun.

I was transferred to the recovery room, where I received additional medications. My parents and Tarun joined me in the room, and they were overjoyed.

Nurses came in and told me that my parents were ecstatic outside, sharing sweets with everyone. I couldn't stop smiling, and I felt immense happiness knowing that my baby had arrived, making us a family of three.

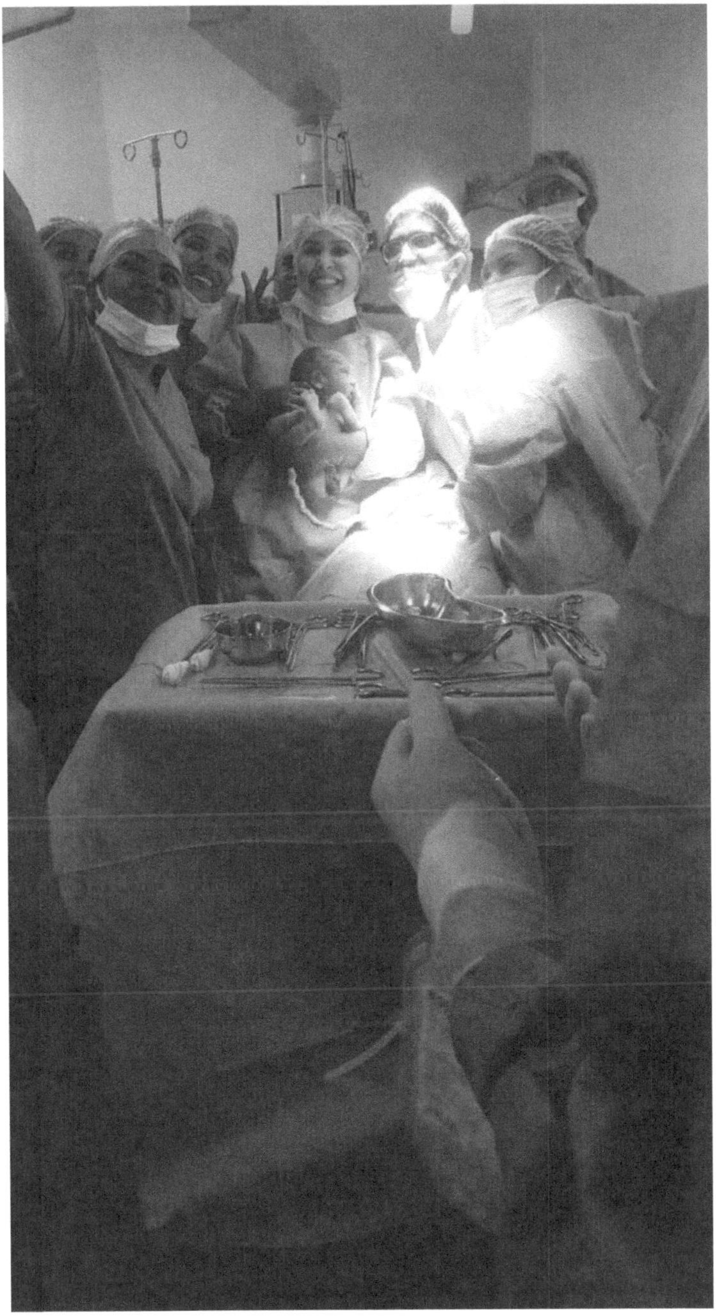

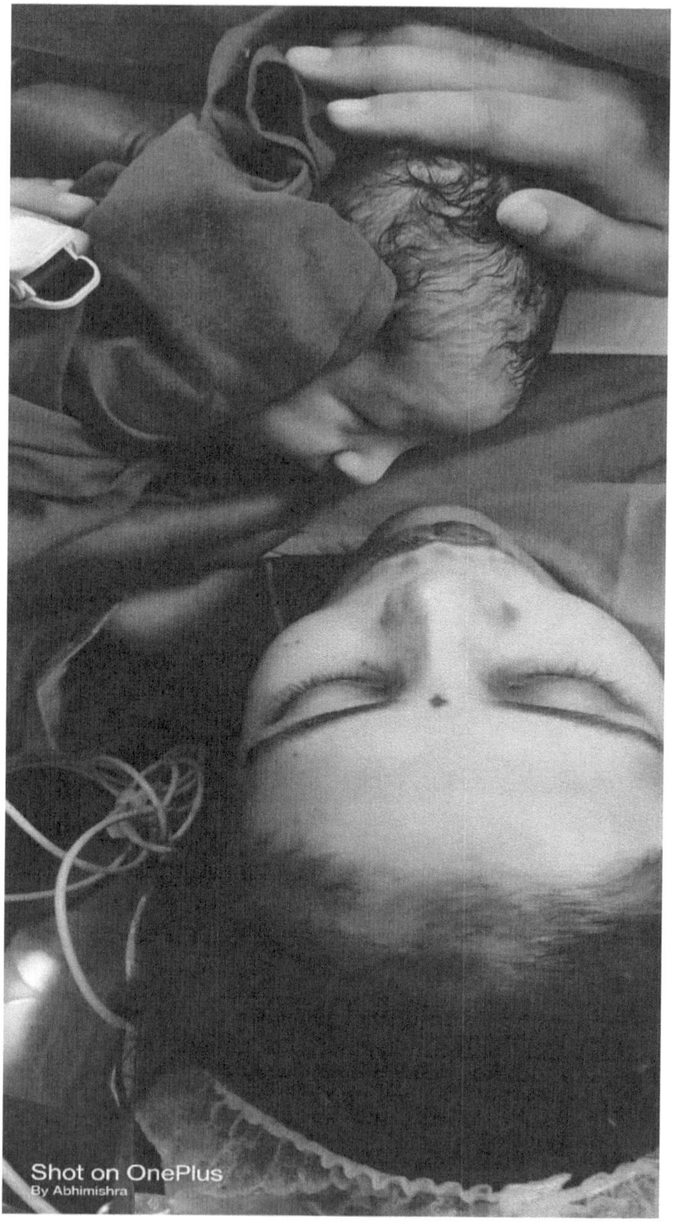
Shot on OnePlus
By Abhimishra

I was given a cozy blanket and monitored closely. The nurses eventually asked me to move to my room, and I was shifted to room 208.

***

My 200th Delivery

As the clock struck 9 pm, I was informed that my delivery marked the hospital's 200th successful delivery for the month, and this was cause for a grand celebration in the operating theatre. It felt like we were setting a new record by achieving the highest number of deliveries in a single month, and surpassing the 200 mark was a remarkable feat.

I began to grasp the significance of the moment. Various individuals came into my room to offer their congratulations. It seemed like everyone knew that my baby was the 200th addition to the hospital's delivery records, and this achievement was widely recognized.

The following day, a significant setup was arranged near the canteen for the Onam celebrations, and I was invited to cut the cake for this special occasion.

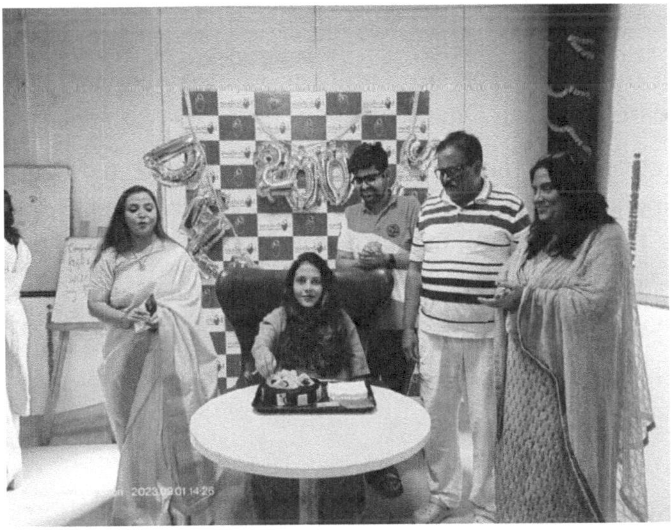

It was heartwarming to hear the hospital's marketing representative acknowledge, "In addition to the joy you've brought to your family, you've also brought happiness to our hospital family. It's because of you that we've achieved this milestone of 200 deliveries."

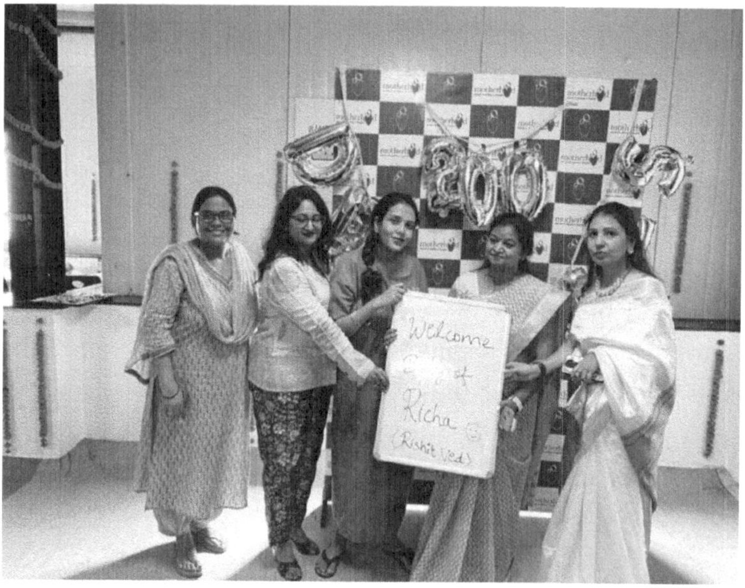

Both my doctor and my family were also honored, and we were treated to an Onam lunch.

Moreover, the hospital generously provided us with gift hampers, discounted our room rent as a token of appreciation, and offered complimentary meals on the day of our discharge.

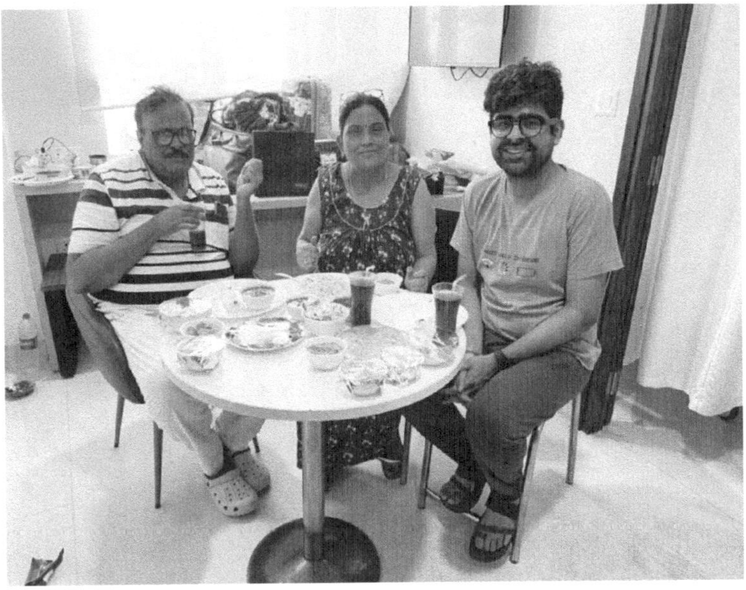

The entire delivery experience was memorable for both the hospital and me. I still can't believe how smoothly everything went. The hospital's team delivered all the value-added services included in the package, such as photography, capturing my baby's feet, and decorating our car.

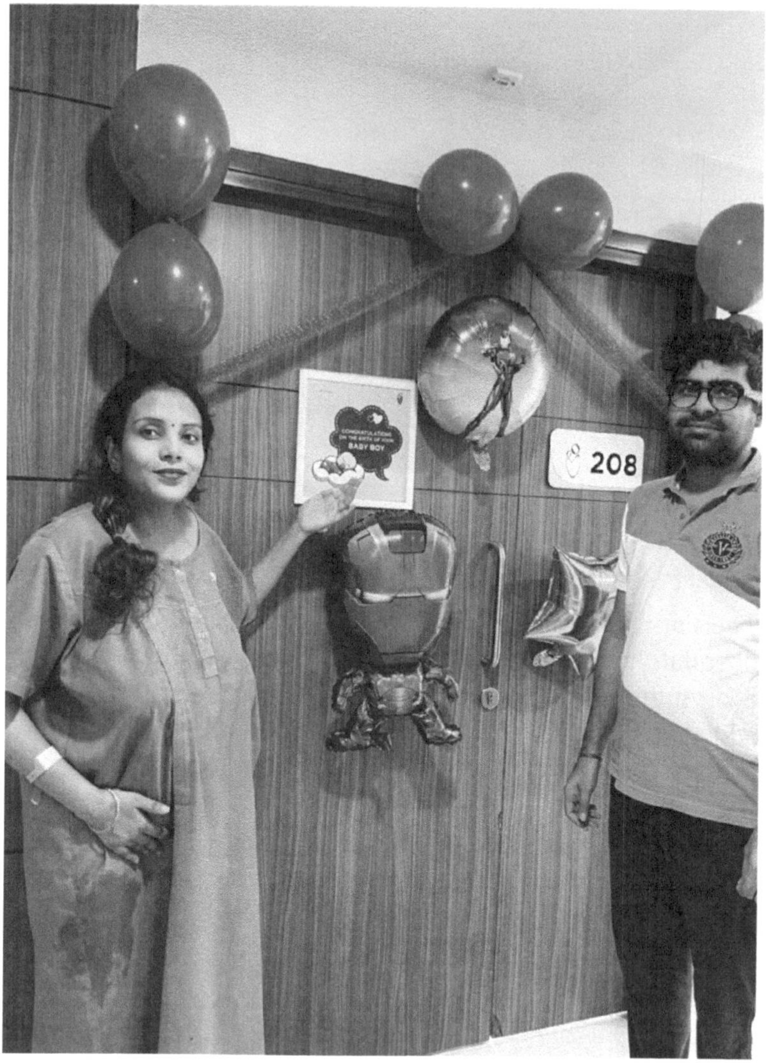

Jyoti and Charu brought the cake again on the discharge day.

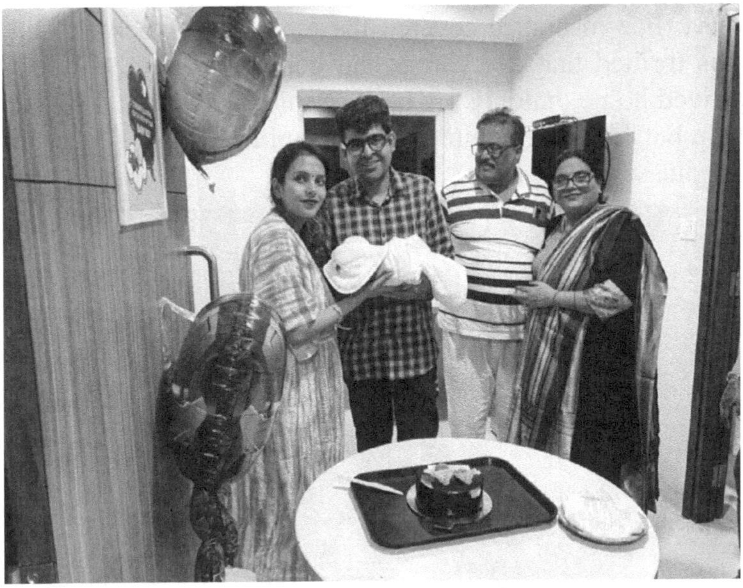

Jyoti provided a special gift package from Himalaya on the 200th delivery.

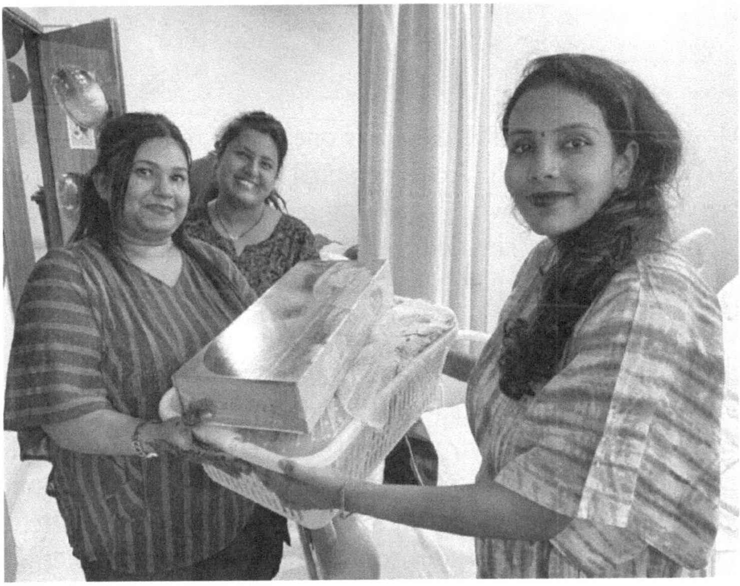

My office insurance covered the remaining expenses, and I was thrilled that everything had gone so perfectly. When I arrived home, holding my baby Rishit in my arms, I couldn't help but feel overwhelmed with happiness. This is what true happiness looks like.

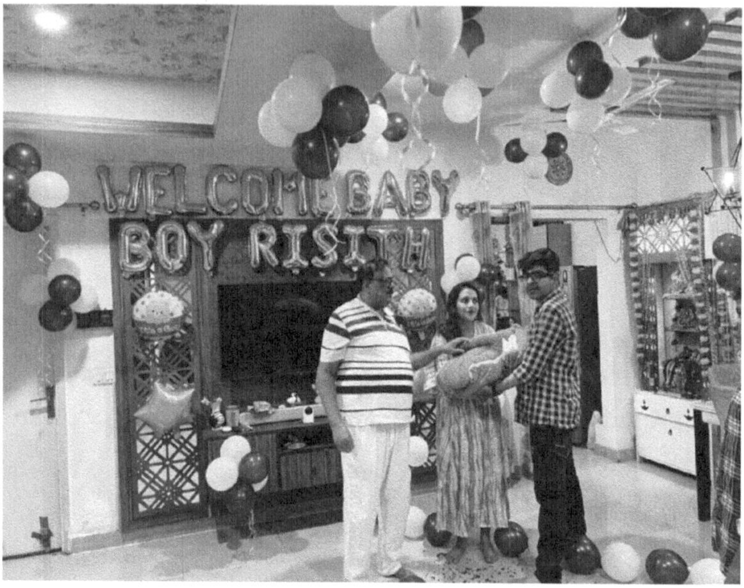

Motherhood Noida stands out as one of the finest hospitals in Noida for childbirth. I can personally vouch for this, given my initial anxiety when selecting a hospital for the delivery of my first child. The dedication exhibited by every member of the Motherhood Noida staff is truly remarkable.

My delivery was overseen by Dr. Manisha Ranjan, a remarkable professional who embodies politeness, genuineness, and excellence. She adeptly managed my complications, instilling confidence in me until the very end. Dr. Manisha has an incredible ability to remember her patients and is the epitome of perfection in her field. I wholeheartedly recommend her if you desire a comfortable, enjoyable, and stress-free pregnancy experience.

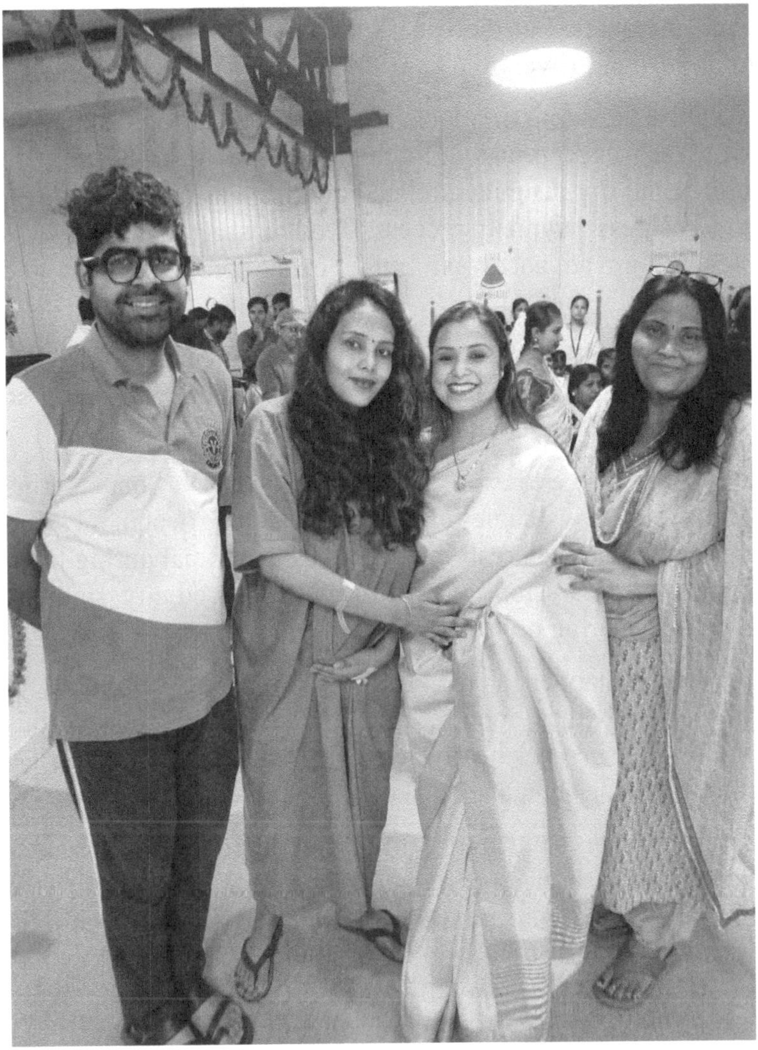

Beyond the doctors, the duty doctors and nurses create a comforting environment. Dr. Parul is incredibly sweet and empathetic, understanding the challenges patients face. Sister Chandni patiently addresses all queries. Among the nursing staff, Neelam ji is exceptionally friendly and helpful. Sister Nandini in the NICU is another example of their dedicated team members, but the list is extensive, and it's challenging to do justice to everyone.

Notably, the admission incharge, Charu, and Ipop Counsellor, Jyoti, are exceptional individuals. Charu took the time to address all our insurance-related queries, ensuring a seamless and cashless payment process. Jyoti ensured my suite was prepared in advance, exhibiting exceptional foresight and dedication.

I want to mention the marketing team member Md Vishal as well for organizing everything in the hospital and being so courteous.

I would also like to express my gratitude to Dr. Sonia Verma, who provided valuable guidance on latching techniques and taught me various breathing exercises beneficial during labor. Her Lamaze sessions significantly improved my stamina, even considering my asthma.

My baby happened to be the 200th one delivered at Motherhood that month, and the team celebrated this milestone in a heartwarming manner, arranging a complimentary lunch and cake-cutting ceremony.

I will forever be thankful to Motherhood Noida for their exceptional service and unwavering efforts. From the entrance guard who assists with your arrival to the billing department ensuring a smooth transaction, every member of the team is wholeheartedly committed to ensuring every mother experiences the most comfortable delivery possible.